*The*
# POWER
*of*
# CHŌWA

*The*

# POWER

*of*

# CHŌWA

Finding Your Inner Strength Through
the Japanese Concept of Balance and Harmony

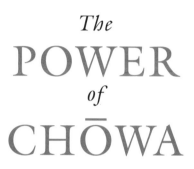

## AKEMI TANAKA

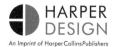

HARPER
DESIGN
An Imprint of HarperCollinsPublishers

Previously published in the United Kingdom in 2019 by Headline Publishing Group.

HarperCollins books may be purchased for educational, business, or sales promotional use.
For information please email the Special Markets Department at SPsales@harpercollins.com.

Published in 2020 by
Harper Design
*An Imprint of* HarperCollins *Publishers*
195 Broadway
New York, NY 10007
Tel: (212) 207-7000
Fax: (855)746-6023
harperdesign@harpercollins.com
www.hc.com

Distributed throughout the world by
HarperCollins *Publishers*
195 Broadway
New York, NY 10007

ISBN 978-0-06-300748-2

Library of Congress Cataloging-in-Publication Data has been applied for.

Printed in Thailand

First Printing, 2020

*To Rimika and Richard*

# Contents

# Part Two: Living in Harmony with Others

# Part Three: Balancing What's Most Important

Dear reader,

My name is Akemi Tanaka, and in this book I'd like to share with you a traditional Japanese approach to finding your balance: *chōwa*.

My name, Akemi, means "bright and beautiful." Tanaka, my family name, means "in the middle of the rice fields," which is fitting as I was born in rural Saitama, part of the now vanished province of Musashi, in a small country town on the outskirts of Tokyo. My family are the proud descendants of high-ranking fifteenth-century samurai who fought alongside the warrior-poet Ōta Dōkan, the architect of old Edo Castle, now part of the Tokyo Imperial Palace.

After a traditional upbringing, I studied Western etiquette at a finishing school in Tokyo before studying at university in Saitama. It was an exceedingly busy time—I was studying English literature and training to be a teacher, and in the evenings working at a Ginza cinema in the bustling capital. There I met my first husband, a young doctor from Japanese high society. I mixed with diplomats, company presidents, and members of the Imperial Family. I was schooled in the art of the tea ceremony and was fascinated by the formal codes of Japan's elite circles. It was a great adventure, like *My Fair Lady*.

I had my doubts about married life. I found myself doing all the little things that have served to keep women out of public life for generations—cooking, cleaning, repairing clothes. I also found myself thinking how I might find the courage to change things for both me and my baby daughter, but in the end, change took me by surprise. My husband and I separated. The divorce left me a social outcast. Divorce was rare and single-parent families were almost unheard of in 1980s Japan. I felt completely taken aback, unable to decide on a course of action or deal with this sudden reversal of fortune.

At this time, I first felt an idea coming into focus. It was a way of thinking I had unconsciously practiced throughout my childhood. It involved being attentive to the balance of my own mind (what was going on with me) and the special balance of a room (what was going on with other people). It stayed with me even when I moved across the world to make a new life in England. This way of thinking, like a sword that had slept at my side but was ready when I needed to wield it, was the wisdom of *chōwa*.

In Japanese, *chōwa* is usually translated simply as "harmony." The Japanese characters in this word literally mean "the search for balance." *Chōwa* offers problem-solving methods that help us to balance the opposing forces life so often throws at us: at home, at work, in our education, and in our personal relationships.

I started to teach others about *chōwa*. I gave lessons to private students in my own home and then to larger groups, to high school and university students. I started accepting invitations to speak on television and radio. The more I taught, the more I felt that the ideas, techniques, and ways of thinking that helped me could be distilled in this concept of *chōwa*. I was convinced that *chōwa* could also help others find their balance.

*Chōwa* is not a mysterious Japanese quality; rather, it is a philosophy, a set of practices that can change our way of thinking about ourselves and others. It's a way of thinking about the world that can be taught—and learned. While learning this age-old concept requires conscious, mindful effort, *chōwa* can teach us practical ways to approach everyday challenges: how to keep our homes clean and tidy, how to achieve a good work-life balance, how to find a love that lasts. *Chōwa* teaches us how to handle other challenges too: how to deal with death and disaster, how to act with the courage of our convictions, how to help others.

Today, I live in London. I have appeared on the BBC and on Channel 4, and have been featured in the *Guardian* and *Daily Telegraph* speaking about issues relating to Japan. I have given lectures at Oxford and Cambridge universities and at the Victoria and Albert Museum in London. I was given a Points of Light award in recognition of the work of my charity Aid For Japan—which I founded after the 2011 tsunami to support orphans of the disaster—by the former Prime Minister of Great Britain, Theresa May.

I hope you will find some of the lessons in this book as useful as I have. While I might once have taken them for granted, the more I've shared and taught about my culture, the more extraordinary I have found the lessons I am about to share with you.

*Akemi Tanaka*

Please visit my website:
akemitanaka.co.uk

Follow me on social media:
Twitter: @akemitanaka777
Instagram: @akemitanaka777
Facebook: facebook.com/powerofchowa

# Introduction

> "Two pilgrims find themselves walking down a long road. One of the pilgrims is wearing a wide-brimmed straw hat. The other is not. It is a scorching day. The sound of the cicadas is deafening. Neither of the pilgrims says a word to one another. They walk slightly apart, giving each other space for their own thoughts. After a few minutes of keeping one another company, the pilgrim wearing the straw hat takes it off and ties it to his pack. They keep walking, side by side."
>
> —Inspired by *Bushidō*, Nitobe (1908)[1]

## What is *chōwa*?

I have always thought that the English word *harmony* had a slightly false ring to it. For me, it calls to mind beaming smiles and 1970s "flower power" slogans, dusty porcelain angels on the mantelpiece of an elderly relative, or the beauty pageant contestant who says she prays every night for world peace.

From religion to relationships, it makes me think of an illusory, heavenly ideal—not something that many of us aspire to achieve in this world.

The Japanese word *chōwa*, by contrast, although it can be translated as harmony, is about something far more practical. It is a way of life. It is something that you can actively do. It would be more accurate to translate *chōwa* not as harmony but as something more like "the pursuit of harmony" or "the search for balance."

In Japanese, *chōwa* is written like this:

---

調 和

*chō-wa*

The first character, *chō*, means "search."
The second character, *wa*, means "balance."[2]

---

*Chō* is a simple character, but it has many layers. *Chō* can be used in a literal sense, such as in the verb *to search* when one is rifling through drawers, and in a metaphorical sense, when one is racking one's brains searching for an answer or for inspiration. The character can be used in another verb: to prepare. Here, it means finding order or being ready for an upcoming challenge. Finally, like harmony, *chō* has a musical sense. Think of an orchestra tuning up—the Japanese word for this is *chōgen*, which literally means "readying one's bow." The *chō* character is intimately related to this kind of tuning: it means a gradual series of small modifications or adjustments as we search for the right note, until we find that we are in tune.

*Wa* also means "peace." This can be a state of tranquility and stillness—think of a peaceful atmosphere or a calm sea. Or, when used as a verb, it can refer to a deliberate act of bringing peace, or balancing two or more opposing sides—whether people, forces, or ideas—so they work better together. As a verb, this character is used in an active sense—not just *peace* as a noun, but as an act of softening, moderating, and relieving. Finally, the *wa* of *chōwa* refers to the country of Japan itself, particularly traditional Japan. Japanese clothes are *wafuku*, Japanese style is *wafū*, and *washoku* refers both to Japanese food and a balanced diet. This same *wa* is found in *Reiwa*, the era that began in Japan on May 1, 2019 when the current emperor, Emperor Naruhito, ascended the throne.[3] *Reiwa* means "beautiful harmony" or "the pursuit of harmony."[4]

If we add *chō* and *wa* together, they come to mean "searching for balance"—in a way that is quintessentially Japanese.

In everyday language in Japanese, we talk about *chōwa* as a noun—like harmony in English—but we also talk about *chōwa* as a verb. It is less musical than the verb *harmonize* in English, and it has a less spiritual meaning. It is more everyday, more relatable, more like "going with the flow." Like anything we learn—such as a martial art or playing an instrument—*chōwa* is something we can practice and become better at.

## The land of *Wa*

*Chōwa* teaches us, above all else, to orient ourselves toward practical solutions. Whether in our personal life, our family life, or in our wider community, *chōwa* is about searching for peaceful ways of finding our balance. It requires us to see our own needs and desires objectively and set them alongside the needs and desires of others to bring about real peace. This approach takes genuine humility. It's about cultivating respect for others while also respecting ourselves.

This way of thinking has, for centuries, been considered quintessentially Japanese. *The Book of Wei*, a third-century history book from Northern China (then called Wei), describes some of the first encounters with Japan, which the Chinese called the Land of Wa. Third-century visitors from China noted in their journals that people from the Land of Wa "bow to show respect to important people. They are friendly and respectful to visitors."[5] Journal entries by the Chinese visitors were recorded as part of *The Book of Wei*. They describe the country's reputation for gift-giving, the Wa people's habit of clapping their hands together in prayer, and their fondness for raw fish—customs that all endure in Japan to this day.

## Our most precious treasure

Around three hundred years later, the Prince of Japan, Shōtoku Taishi, ruled over a divided country. He had introduced a Chinese-style system of modern government, up-to-date agricultural technology, and a new religion, Buddhism. Followers of the native Japanese Shinto religion clashed with this new faith. Shinto—"the way of the gods"—was all about appreciating natural beauty and the ritual worship of the spirits, or *kami*. Buddhism, with its concept of enlightenment and its strong ethical expectations, was really only understood by the educated elite. But Prince Shōtoku was able to bring compromise to his country by imposing a peaceful constitution. Buddhism and Shintoism could be practiced alongside one another.

The first article reads:

---

以和爲貴、無忤爲宗。
人皆有黨。亦少達者。

"Harmony is our most precious treasure, disputes should be avoided. We all have our own views, but very few of us are wise."

—Shōtoku Taishi (AD 574–622)[6]

---

To this day, Shintoism and Buddhism do more than coexist in Japan; they complement each other. Many Japanese people see themselves as Shinto or Buddhist, as neither, or as both. The soul of modern Japan was forged from this peaceful, positive response to what could have led to war and disaster—putting harmony before personal preference or self-interest, even before strongly held beliefs. The maintenance of these two belief systems led to the development of a single culture combining an appreciation for the forces that create and govern our natural world with an ethical commitment to other people.

## Why is *chōwa* relevant today?

Much of what visitors to Japan find so beguiling and attractive about the country can be distilled in the lessons that *chōwa* has to teach us. You may have heard stories about Japanese soccer fans making sure a stadium is spotless after a game, or seen videos of Japanese trains where each and every person, even in the heart of the busiest city in the world, commits to cultivating an atmosphere of quiet and stillness.

Since leaving Japan and making a new life for myself in England, I have seen some aspects of Japanese culture in a new light and have even looked at some with a more critical eye. Yet when I tell people about my culture, I find myself coming back again and again to these simple lessons in finding balance. There are practical things we can all use in our daily lives to help us find our balance.

Today, searching for balance, let alone finding it, is easier said than done. We may feel that we have no time to stop and think. We may feel like we are moving through the world mechanically: going through the motions with our families, hoping any difficulties will simply go away; working long hours at our jobs, where we've stopped caring deeply enough about the people we work with, without giving enough time to ourselves or our loved ones; frantically buying things in the hope that they will make our lives a little easier, that they will bring us a kind of "instant balance"; trying to forget the effects our choices have on our natural world, choices that are disturbing the stability of the planet itself. It is high time we checked in on one another, that we all took a deep breath and introduced a little quiet into our lives. Only then can we take a proper look at what is going on with us—and what is going on with those around us. The *chō* of *chōwa*—to search or to prepare. This is the first step in finding our balance.

And then there's the *wa* of *chōwa*: a way of bringing about "active peace." At the beginning of this introduction, I talked about harmony as a noun. It is when we see harmony as a far-off state, a concept or an ideal that it takes on the air of something impossible, even make-believe. But when we see harmony as a verb—living in harmony with ourselves, or living in harmony with others—then we see that there are things we can all do. We come to see that finding our balance—in our places of work, in our personal relationships, in our society—is about actively searching for solutions, never forgetting that we all live on this planet together.

I believe *chōwa* is a way of thinking that we could all benefit from—now more than ever.

Finally, I would like you to remember throughout this book that, as in the parable at the start of this introduction, *chōwa* is a commitment to responding as generously and as bravely as we can to the world around us. It is about being open to others so we can share in their suffering as well as their joy. And it is understanding that we are all on the same journey: the search for balance.

## *Chōwa* waypoints

I don't think that any of the ideas I share with you in this book require much extra explanation. But I'll do my best to explain sometimes rather knotty Japanese proverbs as clearly as I can, and when I do give examples from my life, or share stories from family members or friends whose lives in Japan may seem distant from your own, I'll try to relate these experiences back to something more universal. I will also give you a chance to pause and reflect along the way by asking you questions to consider, or summarizing the ground we've covered together. Let me sum up briefly what this book is all about.

- How to cultivate an everyday state of readiness, flexibility, and endurance to help us find our balance.

- How to engage in a spirit of open-heartedness with others and better manage difficult emotions.

- How small changes in what and how we eat, and how we treat the natural world, can bring balance to our minds, bodies, and souls.

- How to face up to death and disaster, to prepare for the worst, knowing that it will come, and how to pick ourselves back up again.

# Part One

# Finding Your Own Balance

## 第一章

## 自分の調和を見つける

# 1

## Opening Doors

> "In every doorway
> the mud from wooden sandals.
> It is spring again."
> —Issa (1763–1827)[7]

Japan is home to some of the oldest wooden structures in the world, including many traditional houses. While some of these buildings have a certain elegance, they aren't always what you might call beautiful. What strikes me as more uniquely Japanese, rather than a minimalist look or a pleasing *wabi-sabi* simplicity, is the way every room, every item of furniture, is an exercise in forethought, planning, seeking, and maintaining balance—with nature, with the rhythms of family life, and with the harmony of the house itself.

I want to draw some key *chōwa* lessons for you which I've taken from the wooden beams, the *shōji*, paper-screen doors, the tatami floors, and the daily routines that make a Japanese house a home—lessons in living in our homes, as well as lessons in giving back to the places we live in. These may require us to show our gratitude to our homes in ways that might at first surprise you: cleaning the bathroom, making up a room for an unexpected guest, drying your clothes, taking a bath, or coming home.

Some of the key *chōwa* lessons I'd like you to think about in this chapter are:

- **Respect the rhythms of your home.** I'd like you to think about what each space might be asking for, what each daily routine might really mean. By tuning in to what our homes need from us, we can learn to really feel present in our homes.

- **Bring your home into harmony with nature.** *Chōwa* is about accepting the world as it is, which means finding a way to reconcile ourselves with the ebb and flow of time. We have to accept that wear and tear happens. We have to accept that sudden, unexpected disasters may happen. I also offer a few ways you can allow the natural world into your daily life.

## *Wabi-sabi* and *chōwa*—what's the difference?

The Japanese home has fascinated interior designers and architects outside Japan for centuries. Here I don't want to go over old ground, especially as certain concepts—such as Japanese minimalism and *wabi-sabi*—may already be known to some of you. So before I show you around a Japanese home, I'd like to spell out the difference here between *chōwa*—"the search for balance"—and the concept of *wabi-sabi*—flawed, fragile beauty, or natural simplicity.

*Wabi-sabi* • What is *wabi-sabi*? It means fragile beauty or natural simplicity. It is the knowledge that nothing lasts forever and that everything comes to an end. This Buddhist concept has inspired much that is great in Japanese art and poetry, as well as influencing the architecture and design of Japanese homes.[8]

I immediately think of the Japanese writer Jun'ichirō Tanizaki. His short book on Japanese aesthetics, *In Praise of Shadows*, urges readers not to forget the traditional elegance and melancholy beauty of old Japanese houses—he loves the grain in old wooden floorboards, or the sight of rain running across the mossy foot of a stone lantern in the garden.[9]

*Chōwa: searching for balance* • *Chōwa* means the search for balance. Thinking through *chōwa*, both in relation to our homes and throughout this book, helps us to concentrate on the journey, the *act* of balancing. *Chōwa* helps us to see what it might take for us to feel better prepared, even for the very worst, in our daily lives. It takes hard work. It doesn't happen by itself. We have to go out and actively do something to bring balance to our lives. Thinking through *chōwa* leads us to accept that we will never reach the hallowed state of balance, or harmony. We might even say that *any* kind of balance is always a balancing act.

*Wabi-sabi* and *chōwa* do have some points in common. To feel balanced, it is important to see the world as it really is. This may well mean embracing the perfectly imperfect harmony of nature. But I want you to remember that *wabi-sabi* is far from the whole story (even if this loan word is used by some Westerners as a substitute for "Japanese-y"). Particularly when it comes to the more aesthetic ideas behind *wabi-sabi*, we should remember that our attitudes to our home—in Japan, or wherever we live in the world—are not merely about cultivating this Japanese idea of melancholy beauty. After all, we need to actually live in the place we call home.

**Bringing *chōwa* home to you** • As you are being shown around a Japanese space, you might think, "This is all very lovely, but how can I apply these lessons to my own life?"

A house is like a language. It has its own grammar. If my teaching of Japanese has taught me anything, it's that explaining grammar to a non-native speaker is no small challenge. When you think about bringing *chōwa* to your own home, I am not asking you to throw out your routines—whatever you do to relax, express your appreciation to the people you live with, and how you take care of your home. There will be things about your home life that you can't change even if you wanted to: we choose our homes because they are affordable, or because they are close to work, or because they are big enough to house our families.

Neither am I suggesting that you overhaul the design of the home you live in—to replace your carpets with tatami flooring or your windows and doors with sliding *shōji* screens. But I will explain some *chōwa* lessons from the Japanese home. They include learning to be as prepared as we can—for unexpected guests as well as for more dramatic life changes. Because, wherever we happen to live, we are all capable of bringing *chōwa* home with us: to listening more carefully to what our homes need, so they are ready to give us what we need in return.

Please allow yourself to be guided around these spaces, with the knowledge that they might be a little different from the spaces you usually spend time in. I will do what I can to help you bridge the gaps, to help bring the spirit of *chōwa* home to you.

## The Tanaka family home

I am going to invite you to travel fifty years back in time with me to visit my childhood home in rural Musashi province, north of Tokyo. The province no longer exists today. The area where I grew up is now in modern Saitama.

Walking toward the house from the train station, all you can see are fields and more fields. You pass a small farm. It's still early in the year, but you can see from the fronds of dark green leaves spreading across one small plot that the *daikon* (winter radish) has been planted in anticipation of the coming spring. You pass a temple graveyard with an overgrown willow tree. You hear the striking of a gong and two loud claps. Someone is saying a prayer.

Just beyond the temple and the graveyard, you turn up a rough path and approach a large wooden building. On your left are some tumbledown stables. Sitting just outside a hut on your right is a basket of what look like small, fluffy eggs. These are the cocoons of silk worms. The small hut is a silk-worm farm which produces silk for kimonos. You continue up to the entrance of the large wooden building. Its overhanging eaves are covered with *kawara* clay tiles and supported by pillars of dark wood. You climb three stone steps to the entrance. You look for a knocker or a bell, but there is none. Cautiously, you slide open the wooden door and step inside.

*Step up: achieve positive momentum and readiness at the door* • You are now standing in the small *genkan*, or entrance-way. The *genkan* can still be found in modern Japanese apartment buildings today. It's a place for guests to take off their shoes and for the owners of the house to receive visitors. As this is a traditional house, you can see that, on top of a cabinet for keeping shoes—a *getabako*—is a vase containing a sprig of plum tree blossoms. It reminds you that, while it is still cold outside, you can already feel the first stirrings of spring.

You hear a voice from the end of the corridor. As I've been expecting you, I call out, "*O-agari kudasai!*"

This greeting means "please come in"—it literally means "please step up." This is because, when a person enters a tra-ditional Japanese home, they step up from the *genkan* into the hallway. As you step up into the house, you are expected to take off your shoes—in one movement. If you are unused to this, you may end up stepping on the ground by mistake. Over a lifetime this movement becomes second nature.

You notice that all the other shoes in the *genkan* are lined up against the step, facing the door. You do the same, turning your shoes so their toes point toward the entrance. Now you will be able to slide your feet straight into your shoes when it is time for you to leave.

This is a little example of *chōwa* in action: *chōwa* is about being ready each moment to face the next—small acts that prepare us for an uncertain future.

*Make care conscious: "please go safely, and make sure you come back"* • When a family member leaves the house, they say "*I-tte-ki-ma-su.*"

This means "I will go and come back."

The person who remains in the house will say "*I-tte-ra-ssha-i.*"

This means "Please go, and make sure you come back."

There is a heartbreaking tension in this daily ritual—between our desire for our loved ones to return to us and our awareness of the possibility (one that many people find too terrible to imagine) that they may not. If you have ever stayed up late waiting for a loved one to call you or to arrive home after they have been away for longer than expected, you will know what I mean. This ritual signals a commitment to prepare for whatever the world outside throws at us. Since natural disasters are so common in Japan, we have to be ready for the worst. That is partly why we say "please make sure you come back." It is why we keep an earthquake survival bag in the porch of our house and designate a meeting point where the whole family will meet in an emergency.

This is a central message of *chōwa* that will come up time and time again in this book: living in balance with ourselves, as well as one another, is about matching up the things we say and the things we do. The search for balance with our families and in our homes can begin with stating our hopes and fears aloud, making the way we care more conscious.

This is something I have had to think about more recently, now that many of my family members don't speak Japanese. I can no longer rely on these rituals; I have had to think of ways in English to put into words just how lucky I am to live with the people I care about. Sometimes it is difficult. But since you never know what tomorrow will bring, I would encourage you to do the same.

*Tatami: finding our balance at home, finding our balance in nature* • Once you step up into the house, you pass along a corridor. At the end of the corridor is a room with a tatami floor. Setting your bare feet on tatami feels a little like you are walking on dry grass. In fact, tatami is made from finely woven rice straw. The smell often reminds me of tea, partly because tea ceremonies should always take place in a tatami room, and partly because the smell of rice-straw reminds me of *genmai-ha* (brown rice tea). When walking on tatami, people either do not wear anything on their feet, or—as I do—they wear small white traditional *tabi* socks (wearing shoes or slippers is not permitted).

Focusing on the soles of one's feet, placing them on the ground shoulder-width apart, whether sitting down or standing up, rooted to the floor as one breathes, is a common meditation technique. It makes us feel balanced. I think this is one reason it gives such a feeling of peace to walk barefoot, or wearing *tabi* socks, across a tatami floor, just like it does to walk barefoot outside in a field or through a forest.

In my home in London, while I no longer have a tatami room, I do have a small garden. When I want to practice feeling grounded, more connected to the earth, I go outside and practice this simple meditation technique. If you want to feel grounded in your home and more in touch with the natural world, you can do the same. Stand or sit in a quiet space and pay attention to your breath. Try standing outside, in your garden, in a public park, or simply opening a window and letting in the fresh air.

As you inhale through your nose, focus on the feeling of coolness and pleasantness of your breath. You may feel your breath filling your body with vitality and energy from the ground and from the sky.

Exhale slowly through your nose. The exhalation relaxes the body. You may feel the sensation of tension being expelled.

Focusing on breathing in for a slow count of eight, and out for a count of eight, allows you to feel a gradual, natural kind of relaxation. Try to do this for five minutes. It really helps to focus your attention on your breath and on the present moment. As your breath calms and becomes orderly, so does your mind.[10]

*Shōji screens: expect the unexpected* • Let's suppose I have invited you to the Tanaka family home for a celebration. The main tatami room is a large one. Ten people or more could comfortably sit down cross-legged or kneeling to dinner at the large, low table in the middle of the room.

On the ground, several feet apart, are small wooden tracks that run across the room and divide the tatami. These are tracks for the screens, made out of paper and wood, that usually divide this large room into separate spaces for family members. They can be taken off their tracks and stored to suit various layouts of the room.[11]

They are part of the architecture—not just of the home but of Japanese hospitality: a commitment to welcoming an unexpected guest at a moment's notice, or accommodating a family member who might need some space to work late into the evening.

*Shōji* screens have an additional practical function. When the last guest enters the room, for a tea ceremony for example, they will close the screen door firmly and deliberately. It makes a very satisfying thud, audible to the guests gathered around the table. They will have been listening for this sound and they now know that everyone is present. The host will also have been listening for the thud of the closing screen, waiting to begin the tea ceremony.

Expecting the unexpected and responding to life as it unfolds, moment by moment, is what *chōwa* is all about. It starts with how we treat our homes.

Could foldable tables and chairs help you to better use the space in your home? With more of us living in small city apartments, bringing flexibility into our homes allows us to use our space fully, so we can work, sleep, and welcome guests in the same room.

When it comes to furnishing rooms in Japan, balance can literally be a matter of life and death. In an earthquake, a heavy wardrobe could come tumbling down. Over-stacked shelves could collapse. A hanging mirror or picture frame could fall and scatter glass across the room. Even if we don't need to prepare for cataclysmic disasters, I believe that thinking about balance in this more literal way—the weight and the number of objects we have in our homes—can help us deal with more everyday challenges and changes, however unexpected they are. For instance, what would happen if you had to relocate to another city or country tomorrow? It could be for work, for love, or for a long holiday. What would you do with all your belongings? Could you sell them? Give them away? Put them into storage? Today, few of us will live in the same place all our lives, particularly if we don't own our own home, so it's important to remember that lighter objects are easier to move around, transport, sell, and store. Thinking ahead about this literal kind of balance can help us feel less burdened when it comes to making important decisions.

- Where do your close friends live? If some live far away, let them know you are thinking about them. Maintaining connections with people can be as simple as letting them know your home is always open to them. In Japan, *shōji* screen doors, in a spirit of welcome, are often kept ajar.

*Relaxation as a form of readiness* • After taking a tour of the Tanaka family house and having a bite to eat, I would suggest that you stay the night. You may have missed the last train. I would be happy to offer you the use of the family bath. Unlike a Western-style bath, a Japanese-style bath tends to be deeper than it is long. You can sink into the bath up to your shoulders.

To me, it makes perfect sense to bathe every night. It is not only relaxing to take a few moments of calm for oneself at the end of a busy day, but it is also hygienic. Many people in Japan bathe for up to an hour. Taking a bath in the Japanese way traditionally involves washing oneself with a small shower first outside the main bathtub before getting in to soak in the water. The bathroom is typically a wet room with a separate shower and a stool where you can sit as you shower, with a grate in the floor out of which the dirty water can flow. The bath and shower are separated in this way in many Japanese houses. We may even get in and out of the bath a few times to use the small shower, to wash ourselves again, and then climb back into the bath to soak. Once we are finished, we don't pull the plug and let out all the water. Instead we leave it for the next member of the family. The gentle exercise from climbing in and out of the bath is said to be good for the skin.

Bathing at the end of the day allows us to be quiet. We can finally hear our own inner voice. What we are feeling. What we are thinking. When things are noisy outside, we can't hear this voice. In the bath, when we are relaxed, so is our mind. Whatever other people have said to us during the day, there is nothing they can do to disturb this inner voice, this quiet space.

- Could you try some gentle exercises in the bath, such as gentle stretches or massaging the back of your neck with your hands?

- Do you generally read, listen to music, or use your phone in the bath? Try turning off all distractions—even put down your book. Slow down and listen to your inner voice. This is the best way I know of finding my balance at the end of a busy day.

- Try washing at the end of the day, instead of in the morning. This small act of *chōwa*, of going with the rhythm of our day, has more than one benefit—it allows us not to have to rush in the morning and to keep our bed clean. After all, if you go to bed with dirty hair, you will make the pillow dirty.

Tadaima: *practice saying "I'm here now" when you come home* • When a family member returns to the house, they say "*Ta-dai-ma*."

This means, literally, "I've just got here" or "I am here now."

The person who is at home in the house will say "*O-ka-er-i-na-sai*" or just "*O-ka-er-i.*"

This means "welcome back."

We live in a world where we are expected to be always on—responding to emails, checking our phones for messages, on social media, where we are often "friends" with our work colleagues, old schoolfriends, family members, and strangers. The boundaries between home and work and our social lives seem like they have changed forever. But the least we can do is make a proper commitment to being at home when we are at home.

Making this commitment, which we always used to give so easily when we were small—"I am here, now"—can be very important. To a Japanese person, these words sound like a kind of singing, a musical sound that we associate with our family's love for us. We would come home, step out of our shoes, and yell "I'm home," before breathing a sigh of relief and leaving the day behind. It wouldn't be long before we were eating dinner with our family, reading a book, or relaxing in the bath. There is something powerful about this reminder—this daily commitment to being in the present moment—at least when we are at home: "I am here, now."

## Homes in harmony with nature: taking better care of our homes

Today, Japanese people's lives are still closely tied to the rhythm of the seasons, and this is also true of life in the Japanese home. When it comes to finding our balance, we must not forget that this also means being in balance with nature.

*Chōwa*, living in harmony, is not about making a bubble for ourselves and forgetting that we, like everything else in this world, are natural beings. No matter how much plastic we use and how much time we spend in cities of concrete and steel, we are nature, and nature is us.

Like all natural things, we—and our lives—are subject to change.

Like all natural things, we will eventually fade away.

This is not supposed to sound depressing; it's just a fact of life. Accepting this can help us accept the rhythms of nature— and the inevitable wear and tear that happens to our homes. I'd like to show you what *chōwa* can teach us about living in balance with the natural world and paying more attention to what our homes really need from us.

The fact that Japanese homes are largely made out of natural materials—paper, wood, and packed earth—reminds us of these simple but important truths. If you look more closely at the *shōji* screens in the Tanaka family house you will see that, although the house is old, the paper screens look brand-new.

The paper in the screens is usually changed once a year, on the December 30 or 31, before the start of each new year. When I was small, I would love going about with my mother and my aunt, helping to change the screens in my uncle's house. I would punch my hand through the paper, leaving a hole where my fist had gone through, the torn edges curling like white flames. The paper was replaced in time for the New Year celebrations and the house would be left feeling rejuvenated—a natural clean slate.

*Taking care of our homes, inspired by Shinto (the way of the spirits)* • As you walk around the Tanaka family house, you'll see that the wooden corridors are spotlessly clean and so shiny that you can see your reflection in the dark wood.

Some of the methods that Japanese tidying-up guru Marie Kondo has taught readers around the world—folding clothes, organizing one's home, discarding or giving away what you do not need—have been passed down through Japanese families for generations.[12] I think one of the reasons why tidying up, the Japanese way, has become so popular is our often unspoken connection with the natural flow of things: there is an intimate relationship between cleaning our homes and finding our balance. The act of keeping one's home clean is a way of tuning in to the rhythms of nature.

The traditional Japanese religion, Shinto (the way of the gods [or the spirits]) includes the belief that *kami* (spirits) exist in everything in nature—rain, mountains, trees, rivers. This extends to human-made objects in our homes. Being aware of the spirits in the items we are cleaning, thinking of these items as having their own existence, their own needs, makes us mindful of the care they require from us. Even inanimate objects, from fans to shoes, chairs to cars, may have a *kami*—after all, everything we own came, at one point, from nature. Even items made out of plastic or steel are the work of human hands. Shintoism teaches us that all things, human-made and natural, have an inherent value.

Whenever I clean my *kiri-dansu*, the wooden chest of drawers I keep my kimonos in, I often say, "Thank you for coming from Japan with me, thank you for providing me with such good service."

- Do you have any items you use regularly—an armchair, a desk, a watch—that you would like to express your gratitude to for the years of service they have given you? I wonder if expressing your gratitude would encourage you to take better care of the objects—such as finally getting around to having your favorite armchair reupholstered?

- How could you take better care of the natural materials in your home? Do you know what kind of wood your dining table is made from? What are your bed linens and cushion covers made out of? Being more mindful of the materials that surround us not only makes us better able to care for them, but also makes us more grateful to the objects that give us such excellent service.

*Recycling and reuse in the home* • Doing right by the materials in our home also means using them for as long as possible, serving them so they can live out their lifespans healthily and happily. I always feel a twinge of sadness at Christmas in the UK when I see all that wrapping paper ripped off and thrown aside, or stuffed into black trash bags, especially as it has only been used for one day. I always think "*mottainai*"—what a waste.

In Japan, gifts are sometimes still wrapped in a silk patterned cloth called a *furoshiki*. Traditionally, these cloths have many uses. They are used to wrap clothes, which can then be kept neatly folded in a storage cupboard. They are used to carry things (they were once as common as bags or satchels are in the West). They can be used to carry vegetables, bags of rice, lunch boxes, even small infants. When it comes to wrapping gifts with *furoshiki*, after the person receives the gift—which they would usually open privately at home, not in the presence of the giver—they would make sure that the *furoshiki* was returned to its owner so they could use it again. Wrapping a gift in cloth, as well as being an elegant way to give someone a present, is ecologically friendly.

Even if you don't invest in a *furoshiki*, perhaps you could still practice the spirit of reuse the *furoshiki* teaches us by taking a little more care over the paper your gifts are wrapped in, so you can use it again. When wrapping gifts, if you do so carefully, without using sticky tape but string or ribbon instead, it encourages others to reuse the wrapping paper too.

*Taking care of our homes to show gratitude and love* • Inspired by Shintoism, there is a belief in Japan that seems to capture an important *chōwa* lesson in balance: that taking care of our homes is a kind of bargain, if you like; the better care we take of them, the better care they will take of us.

I remember my grandmother telling me that there was even a *kami* in the toilet. If you clean the toilet, she would say, the god of the toilet will be sure to grant you good health, and maybe even good fortune. Not only this, she would say, but if you make the toilet really, really clean, you will grow up to be beautiful. Her lesson was: "If the spirit of the toilet is happy, you will be too."[13]

Cleaning our home makes us feel closer to the ones we love. The people who teach us to clean are often the people who teach us everything we know about life—our mothers, our fathers, our grandmothers, our older siblings. Keeping my own home in some kind of order makes me feel closer to the people I love, both the living and the dead.

*Cleaning our homes to find family balance* • In Japan, many people believe that when the spirit of the house is happy, you are more likely to be happy too. At least that's what my mother used to tell me when I neglected my chores.[14]

However, I differ from my mother. I place much more emphasis on including the rest of my family in cleaning. I find cleaning both invigorating and calming, but that does not mean I should do all the work myself. Cleaning can be a way of bringing more of a sense of balance to our family too—by making sure we are all doing our bit for our home. These days, it's usually just me and my husband in our home, but he pulls his weight too!

*Taking care of our homes as a way of giving thanks* • On September 1, 1923, my grandmother was invited to a friend's house in Tokyo. She was talking to her friend, rocking her baby in her arms—the baby was my mother's older brother, who just wouldn't go to sleep—when suddenly the ground began to shake. My grandmother had experienced an earthquake before, but nothing like this. The whole house shook uncontrollably. Before she knew it, she couldn't see anything. The roof had fallen in. Injured by falling debris, she lay on the ground, unable to move. Everything continued to shake. She clung to her child. This was the Great Kantō earthquake of 1923. Over 100,000 people were killed. My grandmother and my uncle barely made it out alive. When they emerged from the wreckage, many homes had been completely destroyed. Homes made of wood and paper burn fast and, in the fires that broke out after the earthquake, many homes that had been lovingly tended for generations were gone in an instant.

On March 11, 2011, I heard the news of the earthquake and tsunami that had struck Tōhoku in the Northeast region of Japan. It wasn't until later in the year, when I was setting up my own charity to help the survivors, that I visited the temporary accommodations that had been set up for those who had been displaced by the earthquake, the tsunami, and the meltdown at the Fukushima Daiichi nuclear power plant. One of the most upsetting things for the families I spoke to who had lost their homes in the disaster was not being able to clean themselves properly. Dry shampoo is unpopular today in Japan because it reminds people of these desperate times. No one minds taking a few extra minutes each day to wash properly. They know how lucky they are to be able to do so.

Learning from disasters is another lesson in *chōwa*—in sharing other people's pain as well as their joy. The frequency of such disasters reminds people in Japan, even if they haven't directly experienced a disaster themselves, how lucky they are to be able to keep their homes in order. So I practice keeping my house clean in gratitude for my good fortune, to honor the everyday luxury of a tidy home.

## *Chōwa* lessons:
### finding your balance at home

Making your care more conscious

- Do you have a family custom for leaving your home and arriving home?

- Do you wish you could express your love and gratitude to your loved ones more often?

- Are there any small things you could do (such as keeping a flashlight near the door in case of a power outage, or printing a sheet of emergency numbers and placing it where the whole family can see) to help your household be prepared for anything?

**Cleaning your home to find personal and family balance**

- What was your attitude toward cleaning when you were young? How did this change as you got older?

- Who taught you to clean and tidy up after yourself? A parent or grandparent? A sibling? A partner?

- What happens if you try to think of the act of cleaning as a way of honoring the person who taught you how to do it?

**Your home in harmony with nature**

- Like the sprig of plum blossoms you saw when you entered the Tanaka family house, why not place a vase of seasonal flowers in your hall to welcome you and your guests?

- There are many fun ways to find our balance with the natural world. When I was younger, my sister and I would practice an annual tradition called *momiji gari*—hunting and collecting beautiful fallen leaves. Could you go on your own *momiji gari* expedition? What would you collect?

# 2

# Playing Our Part

> *"The unsung pillar has the power to hold up the house."*
> —Japanese proverb

Mother. Father. Wife. Husband. Daughter. Son. Today, the parts we thought we were born to play in our families are changing before our eyes. Many of these changes feel like changes for the better—for example, more and more of my friends are sharing childcare responsibilities equally, and it has become a lot easier for women to achieve a balance between a busy career and raising a family. But for some people it is still hard to manage all the demands modern life places upon us, to reconcile our true selves with our responsibilities to our families.

*Chōwa* can help us manage these contrasting responsibilities. Family harmony in a traditional Japanese sense means asking ourselves, "How can I serve?" It means doing our best to complement one another in the roles we play and the things we do. It means seeing ourselves as part of a larger whole. But while I learned a great deal from my parents about parenting and my responsibilities to my family, I've learned a great deal more from living in two countries—England and Japan—about bringing fun and flexibility to family life, as well as being realistic about what I can expect from myself. It's a balancing act I only really began to learn when I raised a daughter myself.

Some of the key *chōwa* lessons I'd like you to think about in this chapter are:

- **Think of the parts you play in family life as a balancing act.** Living as part of a family is about learning to fine-tune our sometimes too proudly guarded roles and responsibilities, to place a little less emphasis on what's expected of us and more on what we can realistically give.

- **Find harmony in family life.** It is more than possible to have fun with the roles we play—to bring a spirit of *chōwa* to our relationships, to go with the flow a little more, while still honoring where we've come from. It may help if you replace the words *compromise* and *sacrifice* with how we can complement and care for one another as family members.

- **See each other, and yourself, more clearly.** *Chōwa* teaches us to be more mindful about the demands we place on each other, but we also need to learn how to take a break ourselves. When things are at their most challenging, we must learn to take a step back, to practice seeing ourselves objectively, to check in on our own personal balance—something we can forget to do in the midst of family life.

It isn't always easy living with other people, no matter how much we love them, and sometimes we need some space to work out what we can do to change things for the better.

## The house where I grew up

While I spent a great deal of my childhood in and around the Tanaka family home, I did not grow up there. It belonged to my uncle and his family. As he was not the eldest son, my father did not inherit the house, the land, or any of the Tanaka fortune; in accordance with tradition, this all fell to my uncle, the first-born son. To talk about *chōwa* and the family in a more everyday sense, I will have to take you elsewhere...

When you wake up early in the morning in the Tanaka family home, quietly fold away your futon, walk back along the corridor, and slip on the shoes you left in the *genkan* last night. Slide open the door and step outside, shutting the door gently behind you. Walk back along the road, past the overgrown graveyard, along a broad road with misty paddy fields as far as the eye can see.

After a few minutes of brisk walking, you once again pass the small farm. This is where my maternal grandmother lived, and where my mother grew up. A little farther along the road, you come to a smaller two-story wooden house, the first in a row of similar looking houses around 200 yards or so apart.

This is where I grew up.

## Finding a balanced sense of self

In families, we are often faced with seemingly impossible choices. We want to be ourselves, to achieve our full potential. We often feel that as parents, or partners, we have responsibilities, a certain role to play within the family, whether it is "the strict disciplinarian" or "the one who organizes things." Sometimes we feel like we are the only person holding everything together. The energy it takes to keep up this performance can make us feel like we are preventing ourselves from being true to ourselves. Yet these responsibilities feel necessary—somebody has to reinforce the rules, tidy up, bring balance to the home.

I want to introduce you to a word in Japanese that captures this sense of balance we all strive for, whatever kind of family we live in:

---

自分

*jibun*

These characters mean "the self-part" (in the sense of "one part of a larger whole").

---

These characters contain what feels like a very *chōwa* message: that whatever we do, we do in the context of our relationships with other people, as part of a delicate balance we are constantly negotiating with others. Especially within our family, we find ourselves playing a particular role. If our families were different, the role we played would also be different. In a way, *jibun* allows us to reflect on both meanings of the word *part* in English: we are all "parts" in the sense that we are a part of a whole. We are also all playing a part—like an actor playing a role.

I think this Japanese word for *self* can help us to think about finding balance in our family relationships. Today, there is much emphasis on how to be true to ourselves. But thinking of ourselves as *jibun*, the "self-part," teaches us that the divide between our full selves and the "part" we play (that is to say, our role in our society or family) is not as black and white as we sometimes think. What is the self, after all, if not a constant dance between what we owe to others and what we owe to ourselves? It is the lifelong struggle to fulfill our duties to one another without compromising our playfulness and our spontaneity toward them.

What *jibun* can also show us is that the self can be more than this. The self is not just part of a larger whole. It can be a harmonizing force in a sometimes fractured whole.[15]

*Outward signs of inner commitment* • Along with many other children of my generation, I was brought up in line with a strict code of discipline. The character for discipline looks like this:

---

躾

*shitsuke*

This character combines the symbols for: body, posture, or attitude (身) and beautiful, correct, or suitable (美).

---

We will come back several times to the ideas behind this character. It is closely intertwined with the idea of *chōwa*. While you cannot see a person's attitude, you can see the discipline of a person's mind by the way they carry themselves and by their words and deeds. Our bodies—whatever we do in the world—should reflect our minds. We only show other people the quality of our character when the things we do, and what we say or think we'll do, are in harmony.

You are what you do. Turning up to appointments on time, coming home on time to be with your children, making time to catch up with old friends—the sum of your actions, what you actually do, is what determines your character, more than what you say or plan to do.

*Challenging our children* • Imagine that I've invited you into the house where I grew up, the more modest home down the road from the Tanaka family house. You take off your shoes in the entrance and place them just before the step into the house itself, as you did in the larger house.

When you step up into the wooden corridor, you come face to face with my father's favorite hanging scroll. It depicts a tiger carrying a cub in its mouth. Below the image on the scroll are three characters, our family motto: "strength, brightness, and beauty."

| 強く | 明るく | 美しく |
|---|---|---|
| *tsuyoku* | *akaruku* | *utsukushiku* |

The image on the scroll is a scene from a popular folk story. A tiger carries his cub to the edge of a cliff. He slowly releases his jaws, sending the tiger cub tumbling over the edge. If the cub is not able to crawl back up, she is not strong enough to survive.

I am well aware that this image and sentiment are shocking. But back then, when it came to raising girls in particular, my father went against the grain in teaching us to be more than just "bright" and "beautiful"; he taught us to be strong too. He prepared me for times when I would have to face challenges with my head held high and show no fear.

Challenge can be a positive thing. We don't have to treat our children as harshly as the tiger does in this traditional story. My father certainly put me and my sister through tests—locking us in a cupboard when we answered back, for example—that I would never put my own daughter through. But challenge doesn't have to be given in that spirit. It can be a positive thing. Origami, for example, the art of traditional Japanese paper folding, takes a few hours to learn but a lifetime to master. While it can be very fiddly, even fiendish, when one is learning how to do it, it is a great skill for young children to learn, as it stimulates both their fingers and their brains, introducing them to complex rules of geometry even as they enjoy themselves.

*Introduce quietness into your home* • There is something lovely about boisterous, happy children, and I do not subscribe to the view that children should be seen and not heard. I'm talking here about cultivating a general atmosphere of quietness in the home. Adults are just as responsible for this as children. Children are excellent mimics. If I lost my temper, I would quickly find my own rash words repeated back at me. I tried to avoid telling my child what to do, and instead, by doing things quietly and calmly, allowed her to observe, to watch and learn, harnessing her ability to copy by quietly setting a good example. Focusing a child's attention on watching and learning is a great way to prepare them for life outside the home (quiet study, playing nicely with others, and so on). When we are living with other people we want our minds to be calm and clear for times when we need to have difficult conversations, resolve arguments, or share moments of sadness, as well as moments of joy, with them. Bringing quiet into our homes is a big part of making the home a comfortable place where we can properly relax and talk to one another.

*Have fun with the role you play* • Constantly telling your children to tidy up, or to do their homework, or to be on their best behavior is exhausting. I remember that my father put a lot of effort into playing the role of the strict samurai father. I remember him so much more fondly when I think about those moments when the mask slipped.

Every year, just before the beginning of spring, we celebrated the Setsubun festival. If you arrived in our house on this day in February, you would hear my mother, my sister, and me yelling "*Fuku wa uchi, oni wa soto!*" *Fuku wa uchi* means "good luck, come inside" and *oni wa soto* means "demons, stay outside."

In Japanese households, it is usually the father who puts on a mask and pretends to be a scary demon. The children and their mother throw handfuls of roasted soya beans at the demon as he tries to escape. After the demon has been expelled, we all clean the house together.

I remember pelting my father with beans as he growled at us. We threw the beans at him as hard as we could. When my father took off his mask, there were tears in his eyes. I thought we had hurt him, but they were tears of laughter—he had been laughing at our determined little faces.

My father played this role—the strict father—all his life. When I think of his sweaty face emerging from behind the mask, I think about the daily effort it must have taken. Here are a few thoughts to keep in mind when we're wearing the mask of our family role:

Try not to get caught up in the role you think you "should" be playing. Whether you are trying to be the partner or the parent you think you "should" be, you have to admit that you are a mix of what your parents taught you and what you learned from others. We all invent ourselves as we go along. We could all do with taking our roles a little less seriously.

Stop being stubborn. We sometimes tell ourselves that it is our job to do something—whether that's managing the household budget, planning trips, or doing the cooking. This can be in a positive spirit of contributing to our families whatever we do best. But we can start to lose our balance as a family when something that started with the best intentions becomes something else entirely: a means not of serving our families but of serving and isolating ourselves: "I'm the *only* one who can plan our holidays properly" or "I'm the *only* one who can look after our money." Getting this balance right—listening to other family members and taking everyone's opinion on board—is crucial to family harmony. If you have to talk to a family member who is refusing to listen, reframing "criticism" as a discussion—"I can understand where you're coming from, but . . ."—can help them to see why they are getting so caught up in their way of doing things. It can even help them see the funny side of their arrogance, pettiness, or stubbornness.

Admit when you are wrong. We spend so much energy on being strict, on being right, on being in control. Don't be afraid to admit to your children when you're wrong or to apologize if you have raised your voice. It is often in unguarded moments that our conventional roles can fall away. It is only then that parents and children face each other as equals—and it is only then that they can find themselves becoming friends.

The samurai spirit: learning to serve our families, learning to serve ourselves • When you think of a samurai, you probably think of a Japanese warrior with a topknot, sword in hand, riding to the rescue like in the famous Kurosawa film *The Seven Samurai*. What you may not know is that the word *samurai* in Japanese comes from the word *saburo*, which means "to serve."

While samurai values are typically associated with men, I'd like to discuss my mother here. As I said, the Tanaka family is descended from the samurai who served the warrior-poet Ōta Dōkan. In samurai times, it wasn't just the men who had to learn martial arts and cultivate the skills to defend their homes—even lead armies if their fathers or husbands fell in battle. Women were also expected, at least in some cases, to take up arms and defend their homes. My mother was raised— if not learning sword-craft and military tactics—with these principles in mind. She was a woman, after all, who once told us that she and her classmates had kept sharpened bamboo spears in the corner of their classroom so that, if enemy forces did invade Japan, they would be ready to meet them in battle and, if necessary, die with honor.

I have tried to carry some of her samurai spirit with me through life, and I'd like to share what she taught me about serving my family—and not forgetting to look after myself too.

Renew your commitment to one another. There were undoubtedly differences between my mother and father. While my mother wasn't always right, many arguments stemmed from my father's small dishonesties or his over-bearing demands. But once a year, on New Year's Eve, we practiced a ritual act of forgiveness, putting aside the "bad things" from the previous year and starting the new year afresh. My father, as the "master of the house," would shake a bamboo stick with white paper from a local Shinto shrine tied to the end of it above our heads in a kind of blessing. This was a Japanese tradition to banish whatever demons, whatever bad things, we were harboring. Each child traditionally bows to their father to show their respect. But what always struck me was that, after my father had dispelled our bad things, my mother would take the stick from him and shake it above his head. What bad things was she forgiving? I would wonder. Some years, my father bowed his head a little lower than usual as she shook the stick above his head, sometimes playfully, sometimes a little more seriously, as if there were quite a few bad things to banish that year. It was an annual act of cleansing, a ritual of renewal and forgiveness.

On New Year's Day we say *"kotoshi mo yoroshiku onegaishimasu,"* which means "please look after me again this year." I think that it is very powerful that each family member says this to each other, not just children to their parents but also parents to children. Our families are not always easy to get along with—and we are not always easy to get along with either—but I found these wordless acts of forgiveness, followed by a verbal commitment to "look after one another," very powerful.

I wonder if it is something we should all practice a little more often—helping each other banish the bad things and renewing our commitment to loving one another.

**Don't be afraid to ask for help.** My mother finds it harder than anyone I know to accept help. But I'd like to think, as we've both grown older, even she has learned to relax a little. This is thanks, at least in part, to my sister and me. I'd like to think we've been good daughters, and whenever I'm back in Japan I give my mother a hand with tasks big and small in the home. She always says she's delighted that I come back more often than her neighbor's daughter, who only works a few hours away in Tokyo. But as well as accepting help from her children, my mother has learned how to lean on her community. The people in her town really take care of their senior citizens. When I visit my mother, I'm always surprised by announcements asking people to be on the lookout for an elderly woman who gets lost sometimes, and people don't mind helping to take her home. I'm always charmed by the sound of the tofu truck coming around to each person's house, bringing fresh tofu to the door. My mother recently became the head of her local senior citizens' association and took on the job of managing their accounts. As well as being a great help to the organization, it is a great help and comfort to her too—it allows her to keep her mind sharp and active and to enjoy the company of other people.

**Share the burden of boring household chores.** *Chōwa* teaches us that research—knowing what needs doing—is the first step to achieving real balance. Whether you live with a partner, a family, or a group of housemates, it isn't uncommon for one person to end up doing more of the housework than others. Make a list of what needs doing. Divide up the chores each week. Rotate the tasks so that everyone gets a taste of what these jobs are like. Remember that there is no such thing as "men's work" or "women's work," only work that needs doing. Sometimes, help with household chores can come from unexpected places. On my last trip to Japan, I brought a cleaning robot back with me to England. My mother, who was at first skeptical—she has never even owned a dishwasher—became very fond of the robot and nicknamed her Kuriko-chan. *Kuri* means cleaning. *Ko* is a typical ending for a girl's name. *Chan* is a suffix we use for boys and girls to make us feel closer to them. I certainly feel close to my little cleaning robot. She is doing a sweep right now of my study in London. As I write, I lift my feet to allow her to eat up the dust bunnies under my desk.

**Fight for your right for a holiday.** My father worked long hours at a shipping company in Tokyo. If his boss decided to stay late at the office, all the other employees would have to stay late too. My father would then be expected to go out drinking with his colleagues, whether he liked it or not, and would come home late almost every evening, only to set off again early the next morning. All of this would have been impossible without his equally hard working, largely stay-at-home wife—my mother. A balance, of sorts, was struck, although not the kind of balance any of us would endorse or aspire to today.

While my mother did so much to support my father, often without a word of complaint, I began to see more of her fierce independence, her samurai spirit, as we got older. The cracks started to show as she started to assert her rights with a little more firmness.

Once her children left home, her samurai spirit started to come out in surprising ways. When we were younger, my mother used to dread family holidays. She was expected to look after my father and cater to his every whim—even carry his bags for him. When my sister and I moved away, she put her foot down. She told him she wasn't going to stand for it, and that for her next holiday, she was going to go away with her friends instead. It was a small act to set right a balance that, for a long time, she felt hadn't been working for her.

Look at your life from another perspective. *Chōwa*, searching for balance, requires us to open our eyes to what's really going on. Sometimes we need to be able to look at our own lives objectively, to ask ourselves calmly, "How do I achieve balance in my life?" Asking the question, let alone knowing the answer, isn't always easy.

There's a Japanese proverb—"a frog in a well knows nothing of the ocean." I think about this when I think about my own experience of challenging relationships and those of my friends.

Sometimes you can feel like a frog in a well. You go about your daily life, knowing that you're not happy, knowing that you need to get out or you will drown. Yet you have no idea how to escape. Like the frog in the well, you hurl yourself at the walls. Perhaps these leaps are small compromises you think will help you escape—or indeed, the sense that things are improving—but each time you find things slipping again. You grow more exhausted each time you try to change things.

Sometimes we need someone to talk to. When you are at the bottom of the well, it can be the hardest thing to call out to someone else. Talking to someone can give us a fresh perspective and can help us see that the balance of our lives is far more disturbed than we thought.

It can even be possible to give ourselves this gift of perspective. Try looking at yourself from above, like the moon or the sun sees the ground below. Step back from yourself and be objective. If you take a few moments to imagine yourself living your life, you will start to notice that you feel calmer and more in control. You have stopped fighting, stopped leaping at the wall like the frog, and started to really see what is going on in your life.

Now ask yourself, what needs to change?

## *Chōwa* lessons:
## finding your balance in your family

- Whether you're male or female, "the organizer" or "the strong one," the "lazy one" or "the practical one," you will contribute much more to your relationships when you become less attached to the roles you have been assigned, or assigned yourself, and think more about how you can complement your partner, family, or friends.

- Forget whatever role you usually give yourself.

- Focus instead on what you can actively do to seek a state of real balance.

- Try softening your roles and responsibility in the home with a little humor. It's okay to let your mask slip.

- What stories do you tell yourself about the kind of person you are? Is there part of yourself which you would like to bring out more?

- What allows you to bring out your inner poet, your inner samurai, your sensitive side?

- Are there ways in which you could delegate work more evenly for a fairer balance among members of your household or your roommates?

- Remember that doing all you can to do what's best for your family can be exhausting—and that often your greatest enemy is yourself.

- Do what you can to fight for your right for a holiday, even if it's just a day off.

- Find allies, both within and outside your family, you can talk to about problems when they inevitably arise.

3

## Balancing the Books

> "Making money can feel like digging a hole with a needle,
> but spending it is like water disappearing into the sand."
> —Japanese proverb

For many of us, money is the biggest source of day-to-day stress and anxiety. There have been times in my life when I had little to worry about financially—when I was able to depend on my family, or my husband, or the profits of my business when I ran an English school in Tokyo. Yet even at these times, I would find myself waking up in the middle of the night, worrying about what would happen if this support fell away or what I would do if my success suddenly faded. There have also been times when I have struggled with money, such as when I moved to England and had to work very hard to make ends meet. But in good times and bad, I have always been most anxious when I have felt I have not been paying my personal finances enough attention. I think this is true for us all. We need a handle on the basic facts to achieve financial balance. How much are we earning? How much are we spending? How much are we saving? What do we really want to spend our money on? What would happen in the worst-case scenario, if disaster struck?

Approaching the way we spend and save with the spirit of *chōwa* (just as we approached our homes and our families) can help us find financial balance. When we start to think of ourselves more like an accountant, with an eye on "balancing the books," we start to feel on firmer ground.

Some of the key *chōwa* lessons I'd like you to think about in this chapter are:

- **Think of saving as a balancing act.** I'll show you that saving can be a matter of keeping a conscious track of your income and expenses. Setting a savings goal can help you put a little more aside each month and can help you consider where each spending decision sits on your personal list of priorities.

- **Own less, give more.** *Chōwa* is about living in harmony with others. This means rethinking our relationship with our things—realizing that it is genuinely easier to balance when we aren't carrying quite so much through the world—and learning how to share our belongings with others to help us build stronger communities in a spirit of sustainability.

## *Kakeibo*—the household finance ledger

Let's imagine we are still in my family's home in Musashi. It's almost midnight. You and I have been talking quietly in the kitchen, sharing a cup of tea. We hardly notice my mother coming into the dining room, sitting down at the low table and taking out a small book. If we were to walk over to her to see what she was up to, we'd find her cross-legged, surrounded by receipts, scribbling numbers in her small book.

If you asked her what she was doing, she'd tell you she was calculating the difference between her income and expenses for the month. This is the foundation, the first step to bringing balance to your household finances. The method, and the journal itself, is called *kakeibo*: the household finance ledger.

*Kakeibo* is the brainchild of journalist and author Motoko Hani. Japan's first famous female journalist, Hani published this system for modern domestic bookkeeping in 1904. *Kakeibo* books have been bestsellers ever since.[16]

## Just another chore?

Is keeping track of our savings just another household chore? Or can it be genuinely useful?

One of the main reasons for keeping a *kakeibo* in Japan is that you never know when your circumstances might change dramatically. The money you save will typically be set aside for surprises, good and bad, such as gifts for marriages or new babies, throwing a party for an old friend who's back in town—or medical bills, paying bills after losing your job or paying funeral costs after the death of a relative. From small change to my father's occasional bonuses, my mother put aside everything she could into the *hesokuri* (emergency pot).

In traditional Japanese households, and still today in many cases, the wife has direct control of the family finances. This includes an allowance she gives to her husband each month called the *kozukai*—a kind of personal budget. This is not intended to be a punishment. There is a lesson here in family balance, in spending decisions taking place in the home, rather than spontaneously by any member of the family. My mother knew exactly what was going into, and coming out of, the family home, and she asked my father to submit his receipts at the end of each week like a good company accountant. As *chōwa* teaches us, when searching for balance, doing our research is a crucial first step.

## *Kakeibo* for beginners

### 1. Organize your income and expenses

- At the start of the month, work out your income (i.e., what you earn) and your fixed expenses (i.e., all essentials, including rent/mortgage, phone bills, utilities, home and personal insurance, season tickets, childcare, gas and other car-related costs or other travel costs, money for food, etc.).

• Calculate the difference between your income and your fixed expenses so you know exactly how much you have to work with this month.

• Think creatively about why you might want to save money—it might be for going on holiday or buying yourself a small present.

• Set your monthly savings goal. Be realistic. Writing it down instills discipline and will help you reach your target (it always helps to have something to aim for).

• Then you can work out your monthly budget:

*The difference between income and fixed expenses – monthly savings goal = your monthly budget.*

## 2. Record your monthly spending

During the month ahead, record what you spend your money on, in categories. You could choose to create an Excel document to do this, but there is something powerful about doing it by hand too, and a good *kakeibo* book makes it easy to do so. They will usually encourage you to record your spending in categories, just as saving apps for smartphones do today, as follows:

Essentials: e.g., food, medical bills, clothes, education for your children

Treats: e.g., drinks, eating out, clothes

Cultural: e.g., books, music, movies, theater, magazines, yoga lessons

Misc: e.g., one-time expenses on repairs, new furniture, or gifts

### 3. Work out how much you've saved

At the end of each month, work out the difference between your initial budget and your total monthly expenses. This will give you your monthly savings. The foundations of the *kakeibo* are as simple as that.[17]

## Balancing what's important: how to save for what matters most to you

Planning how much to save each month, and seeing clearly what you are spending your money on, is more than half the battle when it comes to achieving personal financial balance. But we can easily find ourselves losing control of our spending—picking up a coffee on the way to work every day, for example, or finding it hard to say no to after-work drinks. The foundation of the *kakeibo* is the savings goal: deciding what's important. Consider the following:

- What do you most want to save for?

- How much would you need to save each month to afford it by next Christmas? Or next summer?

- How could you start saving today toward something that is genuinely important to you?

**Don't be afraid to say no.** Decide on a personal savings goal. It might be a holiday with your friends, a deposit on an apartment, or personal luxuries like going to the theater or movies more often. Then when you receive an unexpected invitation or feel tempted to spend—lunch out with colleagues or a night out with friends—you will be able to better assess your own personal balance of priorities. You may end up deciding that your personal goal wins.

*Make yourself accountable for your goals* • At the end of each month, take a look at the savings target you set yourself at the start of the month. Did you hit your target? If not, why? Was it because saving was particularly hard? Why was this? Did you have an unexpected one-time payment (such as a repair, a household expense, or a dinner party that you had to prepare for) that you hadn't factored into your budget?

Be honest with yourself, but don't forget to be kind to yourself too: the carrot (your savings goal, the reason you're doing this) is more powerful than any stick. Keeping a *kakeibo* is like keeping a food diary, and there's no point being dishonest in it. Keeping a record each month will allow you to see where your problem areas lie.

**Share your goals with friends.** There's nothing better to help you feel accountable. Feeling like you have an ally (or a little gentle competition if that's what motivates you) can be a real help and a comfort on your journey to financial balance.

## Accidental minimalism—owning a little less, sharing a little more

The older my mother gets, the fewer belongings she seems to need, and the more she gives away. She has given a few beautiful old kimonos to me and my daughter and given the rest of her things away to friends.

When I moved from Japan to the UK, I had to think very carefully about what mattered to me. I couldn't take everything I owned. In the end, I held on to my kimonos, a few family photos and, of course, my daughter. When my husband at the time and I moved into our new apartment in London, I was struck by the feeling the house gave me. It felt like a clean slate.

My mother and I are "accidental minimalists." When it comes to searching for your own personal balance, thinking about your attitude toward your possessions is a crucial step. If you've ever had to travel with a young child, as well as several bags of shopping, or ever had to navigate the barriers on the London Underground and somehow find your Oyster card without dropping everything you're holding, you'll understand what I mean when I say that when we are less burdened, we genuinely find it easier to balance.

Having a little less tying you down makes it easier to make big life changes, whether it's starting a new relationship, relocating for work, or moving to a new country.[18]

*You don't need objects to compete with other people (or yourself)* • Three sacred treasures are said to have been gifted to the first emperor of Japan from the heavens: a sword, a mirror, and a jewel. But ordinary people have their own "three treasures" too. Following the post–Second World War boom, the vast majority of Japanese households were able to afford a television, a fridge, and a washing machine. These everyday objects made life so much easier and improved the lives of Japanese families immensely. But since then, somewhere along the way, buying new things has stopped being about how they might help us and has become a new way for us to show other people, and ourselves, who we are. A new phone to show how modern we are. A gym membership to show how committed we are to personal fitness.

My advice is not to worry about how to signal things about yourself to others. Get rid of what you are holding on to for the sake of appearances. When you get rid of the gaudy jacket you were never going to wear, or give away the latest novel that you just can't get into, you'll be free of the baggage of competing with other people—and other versions of yourself. Finding our own personal sense of balance involves casting aside not just the things but also the "selves" we no longer need and that we are better off without.

*Share more* • Thinking about our attitude toward our belongings through *chōwa* reminds us that we can't achieve balance by ourselves. Our own sense of balance is intertwined with the lives of other people as well as with the natural world. We are all part of a larger ecosystem. So are the things we own. When we start to include others in the equation of what we own, we start opening ourselves to the idea of a more social economy. We stop thinking of ourselves as islands, but as individuals with things to share, as well as things to borrow, from our communities.

**Active sharing builds communities.** When we stop clinging to what we own and start to let others in on what matters to us, we can start to build a lively community of people with common interests. When I first arrived in the UK, I felt that there was no Japanese community. But little by little, I found myself lending my kimonos, or borrowing equipment for a tea ceremony, or sharing traditional Japanese sweets with my neighbors. When we start to share what's important to us, we grow our extended families and we learn to live in harmony with others.

## *Chōwa* lessons:
## balancing the books

**Your priorities**

• What do you buy regularly that you enjoy? Cups of coffee? Trips to the movies? Drinks with friends? Do you have any habits that, when you really think about it, are not worth the money you spend on them? Instead, could you save the money to spend on something you really love?

• What services do you subscribe to? Gym memberships? Entertainment services? Rank them and see which are most important to you. Are there any you can do without?

**Savings goals**

• What do you want to save for? What would you like to be able to afford in six months, or two years? List some reasons to save money—give yourself powerful reasons to balance the books.

• Use the *kakeibo* method to start making realistic monthly savings goals.

• After a month, see how you've done. If your goals were too challenging, try setting some more achievable ones. If you did a good job in the first month, you may feel motivated to make some deeper cuts. Do what you need to do to move forward with momentum.

# Finding Our Style

> "Taking one layer off
> I sling it over my shoulder.
> Time to change clothes."
> —Matsuo Bashō (1644–1694)[19]

Throughout my childhood, my mother could often be found working from home, repairing kimonos and Western clothes. At a time when I felt that I was casting myself off from my home and my family, my kimonos became an important way to remind me who I was. I got into the habit of wearing a kimono at least once a week in public. I could wear a bright spring kimono on a walk to a country pub, or a light summer kimono on the London Underground. It is such a pleasure to share the elegant, timeless beauty of these clothes with other people. While it takes some forward planning—as it takes a little longer to get around in a kimono—I feel that it is worth the extra effort to surprise and delight my fellow Londoners. I enjoy the satisfaction of getting my outfits just right, and I am proud to keep this tradition alive. I don't spend all my time wearing a kimono, but this traditional item of Japanese fashion has a lot to teach us about style. The kimono itself is inspired by a real spirit of *chōwa*: not only do the colors in each kimono outfit harmonize beautifully with each other, but wearing a kimono is, at its heart, about dressing in harmony with nature and thinking carefully about the effects our style has on others. In a kimono we are more mindful about what we are saying with what we wear.

But the lessons *chōwa* has to teach us about finding our style are not about fitting in, following the rules—or the crowd—or jumping on a new trend to keep up. This isn't what I mean by harmony with others. *Chōwa* can teach us about the power that comes from having confidence and pride in what we really care about. It can be about asking ourselves what makes us feel and look our best. Whatever you wear—you may not have just one style but several—*chōwa* offers ways to think more deeply about rooting yourself in what matters to you, gaining the confidence to share it with others, and learning to feel the sense of satisfaction that comes from embracing who you are.

Here are some of the key lessons in this chapter:

- **Style as a search for balance.** In this chapter I'll share some ideas about how to develop an artistic sensibility toward the colors that make up your wardrobe, to treat style itself as an act of *chōwa*—a way of searching for balance in every outfit.

- **How to root yourself.** I'll be sharing what *chōwa* can teach you about finding your place in the natural world, dressing in harmony with others, rooting yourself in your own personal history and heritage, and asking yourself what is truly important to you.

- **Do what you love, and love what you do.** *Chōwa* teaches us to take stock of our strengths and work with what we have at our disposal—whether that's an item of clothing, such as a treasured hand-me-down, a characteristic, like our determination or creativity, or a passion, such as an enthusiasm for Japanese anime, arts and crafts, or even our love for a certain season or a favorite color. To find our style, we don't need to change our interests, or find new interests that make us more acceptable or more interesting to others. Finding our style is about finding the courage to share what matters to us with others, no matter what our interests are. When we feel comfortable in our own skin, we are much more relaxed around other people.

## Kimonos—1,000 years of fashion

The history of the kimono, which literally means "the thing one wears," stretches back to the elaborate formal wear of Japan's Heian court, over 1,000 years ago. But the kimono as we know it today is most closely related to the *kosode*, a short-sleeved garment popular in the Edo era in the seventeenth century. At the time, what would later become known as the kimono was worn by almost every person in Japan, regardless of age, sex, or class.

A kimono is a full-length dress-like robe, cut in a classic "T" shape. Sleeve lengths vary from long and flowing (for single women) to a shorter cut (for married women). The modern kimono is usually worn by women, but the unisex variant, the summer cotton *yukata*, is popular with men too. Patterns vary greatly. They can be colorful with incredibly elaborate patterns (including famous artworks or lines of poetry) or plain and elegant. They are tied with an *obi* (a silk, cotton, or linen cloth) around the waist. While the cut of the kimono has stayed the same, what used to give away one's social position was the style, the colors used, and the value of the textiles used in the kimono. In the Edo era there were complex rules that dictated which kimono was appropriate for the wearer and the season.

In the 1950s and 1960s, the kimono began to disappear from the crowded streets of Tokyo. People in my mother's generation were far more interested in Western fashion. But in the West, the kimono had already begun to have a major impact on everyday style. Elsa Schiaparelli introduced a more shapeless cut and drape style in the 1920s, consciously inspired by the kimono. Yohji Yamamoto's avant-garde pieces of the 1980s were black and rough around the edges, but still recognizably the same garment as worn by Japanese people in the Edo era.

Today, look at the trend for simple, rectangular-cut dresses and shirts in high-street stores such as Muji and by Scandinavian brands like Cos. The kimono has been remarkably resilient. In Japan, young designers are liberating the kimono still further through exciting new trends and patterns. Recently, it has been popular to dress in your mother's kimono for special occasions.[20]

## Style as a "search for balance"

The act of choosing and wearing a kimono is a constant search for balance, a strenuous but rewarding effort to make sure that all the elements in your outfit are in harmony. I believe some of the lessons I've learned from wearing a kimono apply just as well to modern fashion.

*Finding balance in how you dress, one layer at a time* • If you ever get the chance to read classic works of Japanese fiction such as *The Pillow Book* or *The Tale of Genji*, you'll notice that women often hide their faces behind a fan or conceal themselves behind a bamboo screen, particularly when potential suitors are around. A woman in Japan at this time—during the Heian period, from 794–1185—was admired above all else for her skill and ability in a number of traditional arts: writing poetry, engaging in witty conversation, how she assembled her outfit. At court, sometimes a woman's reputation for choosing beautiful outfits, or a glimpse of her well-chosen color combinations through a *shōji* screen door, was enough to win the heart of a potential lover. The multilayered outfit—of which, believe it or not, the kimono was just one layer—led to women having many options for creating pleasing, and sometimes shocking, color combinations. Men too were expected to create exciting and interesting color combinations to demonstrate creativity and sensitivity, as well as material wealth. When Prince Genji himself turns up to a spring gathering in a beautifully coordinated pink and lavender outfit, he causes quite a stir among the young ladies (and gentlemen) present.[21]

Layer to achieve a quintessentially Japanese style. Building outfits by layering clothing is incredibly practical: a nice blouse, even if it is made from a material that is more suitable for summer, can be worn over a T-shirt or camisole with a warmer jacket so our favorite outfits don't have to languish in our wardrobes over the winter. Layering allows us to tune ourselves much more finely to the weather outside, degree by degree, until we find our balance.

Layer to demonstrate excellent taste. We can show our creativity as well as sensitivity to the seasons by mixing and matching suitable colors and patterns for the time of year.

*Finding practicality and comfort in what you wear* • We don't think often enough about comfort when we are deciding what to wear. In Japan, a tailored look—not too tight, not too baggy—is key. When people ask me if the kimono is comfortable to move around in, they are surprised when I tell them it is perfectly comfortable. While you have to move a little more slowly in a kimono, they are not restrictive—unlike Victorian-style corsetry, for example. Kimonos are a little snug, yes, but not too tight.

Feeling unbalanced and unready can stem simply from not having what we need when we need it: fumbling for a ticket, not having a bag to put important documents or our book in when we are squeezed onto a busy train. Finding our balance in what we wear can be as simple as placing a higher value on convenience and practicality. When I wear a kimono, I can keep my handkerchief and my business-card holder in my sleeve. I can keep letters and even a small book tucked into my *obi*—along with a fan on a hot day.

- What items in your wardrobe make you feel ready for anything?

## Comfort and beauty, in tension

People trying a kimono for the first time often struggle with the *obi*. Usually made of a natural material such as cotton, linen, or silk, the *obi* is tied tightly around the waist. When my daughter was fitted for a kimono, she gave a gasp of resistance as the *obi* was tied around her. The fitter snapped at her: "You've just got to put up with it!"

But while it might seem counter-intuitive, the *obi* is ultimately there for our comfort. A sedentary lifestyle, spent gazing down at a smartphone or sitting at a desk, hunched over a computer, has gotten us into postural bad habits that put a great deal of stress and tension on our back muscles. The trick to better posture is doing as little work as possible with the muscles that we often end up getting to work so hard for us. I always get the feeling, when my *obi* is tied tightly, of a different kind of tension. This kind of uprightness, which once felt quite natural for people who didn't spend their life at a desk, makes me think, "Ah, this is how I'm supposed to be standing."

*Taking care of your clothes* • In Chapter 1, we talked about finding out what kind of care we needed to give the materials that make up our home, whether we're looking after a seagrass rug or a wooden table. We should look after them so that they can better serve us. It's the same balance that we must strike with our clothes.

I frequently find myself talking to my clothes, in my head, making a silent pledge to them. I say, "Thank you for the service you've given me. I promise to try as hard as I can not to make you dirty, and to help you live a long and happy life." The longer we can make our clothes last, the better it is for the planet. The fewer clothes we buy and the more time we put aside to repair old clothes and pay attention to the condition of the clothes we do own, the less we fuel fast fashion and the less we need to buy new items just to have clothes that are clean and in good condition.

After I wear a kimono, I hang it up on a special kimono hanger to air overnight. You cannot wash kimonos often—if you want to, you have to unpick the rectangular pieces, wash them separately, then sew them back together. Whatever we're wearing, a little care can keep our clothes in their best condition.

**Prepare for the day ahead.** Remember, when it comes to harmony with what we wear, that the *chō* of *chōwa* also means "preparation" and "readiness." Get in the habit of checking in on your clothes. You will feel more ready to face the day if, instead of noticing an unexpected crease or a hole in a pair of trousers just as you are about to head out of the door, you have inspected your clothes the evening before.

**Treat your clothes with care.** Don't throw your clothes on the bed at the end of the day or leave them in a pile on the floor. Consider how your clothes feel. Are they really happy to be crumpled up on a corner shelf of an old wardrobe or jostling with one another for space on tightly packed hangers?

## Harmonious style: dressing for the time, the place, and the occasion

When one is dressing in a kimono the traditional way, it is usually necessary to consult an etiquette book that will tell you what kind of kimono is suitable for each time, place, and occasion.

Kimono guide books place a special emphasis on dressing in harmony with the moment:

- time—consider the time of year, the season, the weather

- place—consider where you are going

- occasion—consider whether it is formal or informal or a special event, such as a wedding (and consider the people who are also likely to be there)

The same *chōwa* lessons that underpin the wearing of kimonos—dressing in harmony with other people, with the time of year, and appropriately for specific events and ceremonies—can offer us ideas to bring balance to our wardrobes, whatever we're wearing.

*Time: finding your balance with nature* • There are strict rules that govern the wearing of kimonos, and some kimonos can only be worn on certain days of the year.

When Japanese people wear kimonos, we do our best to be *shizen ni awaseru* (in harmony with nature). I hope you can take inspiration from Japanese kimono design for seasonal colors and patterns to try out yourself.

*Winter*—one usually wears a lined kimono in rich, bright color combinations, sometimes even colors that clash, like dark greens with bright oranges, or Christmassy red with white (such as red flowers or berries in the snow).

*Spring*—colors tend to be light and fresh, such as bright pink with white and green; purple with white; a bright daffodil yellow with a slightly deeper, more golden yellow. In early spring one can wear *ume* (plum blossom) and *sakura* (cherry blossom) patterns. Floral patterns are fine to wear throughout the spring.

*Summer*—people tend to wear kimonos in *usumono* (a translucent fabric). The Japanese summer is very hot and humid, and it is thought that even seeing the icy blue patterns on someone else's kimono—like an ocean wave, rain, or even falling snowflakes—will give the onlooker a refreshing feeling of coolness, like feeling an ocean breeze on a warm day. Summer is also when men and women wear *yukata*, a more casual summer kimono.

*Autumn*—in autumn, kimonos also tend to be made of light fabric. Colors should be reminiscent of autumn scenes—falling leaves or sunlight through the trees in purples, reds, oranges, and yellows.

A word of warning: it is thought to be slightly crass and bad taste to wear, for example, a kimono with a cherry blossom pattern when the cherry blossoms are actually in flower. Rather than being in harmony with nature, this is seen as competing with nature. Nature itself, the real thing, will always win.

I try to get ahead of the game when it comes to wearing clothes for the spring and the summer. My friends laugh when they see me wearing something summery a week or so ahead of the warm weather, but there is something lovely about bringing in the changing seasons for them.[22]

Dressing in harmony with the seasons doesn't mean that you have to go out and buy the latest must-have autumn coat or summer dress. It can actually help you to become more resistant to the roller coaster of fast fashion. Taking our cues from nature can begin with learning to layer using items we already own, not letting fashion magazines decide what you will wear this season. Take in the air outside and think about what item in your wardrobe is asking to be worn today. While this means taking care of your most treasured pieces so you can rotate them seasonally, the effort is worth it for the service they will give you year after year.

*Place—bringing ourselves to whatever we do* • In Japan, we believe that each area of our lives is likely to require something quite different from us, and this is reflected in the way people dress. It is true, of course, that people in the West may dress in a suit and nice shoes for their office job in the morning, and slip into something more comfortable when they come home in the evening, but the divisions between outfits for the different roles we play, and the different places we inhabit, is a little starker in Japan. Workwear is typically more formal. Loungewear is more explicitly made for relaxing in. When I'm in Japan, I tend to change clothes at least three times a day. While this might sound excessive, it isn't uncommon, and clothes are tailor-made for each place we are dressing for:

- Household wear is called *heyagi*. It tends to be loose, baggy, and casual—lounge pants and loose, hooded tops, or oversized comfy throw-on dresses and robes made of a soft material. There are even matching indoor clothes for couples if you want to be especially cute.

- Everyday wear is called *fudangi*. This tends to be practical and easygoing, the kind of clothes you can wear around town or to meet a friend.

- Workwear is called *shigotogi*. Office wear in Japan tends to be classic, and more formal than in Britain and in other Western countries. For men, suits and ties are mandatory in most workplaces (no jazzy ties or pink shirts). Women wear high heels, nice plain knee-length skirts, and tights in neutral palettes.

This might sound a little regimented—and to some extent I think it is. When some people think of Japan, they think of rows of identically suited salarymen waiting for a commuter train, or obedient schoolchildren in uniform, sitting upright and ready to learn. But these stereotypes conceal the more exciting history of ordinary Japanese people's passion for fashion.

In Japan, popular style has always come from the grass roots. It wasn't the case that peasants wore rags and the gentry were the only people to wear gorgeous clothes. Rural families wore cottons and some even wore silk. Even overalls for farm work and the aprons of street vendors were designed and fit for purpose. There was a strong appreciation for beauty, an enjoyment and love for the clothes one wore for leisure, for formal occasions and for work, whatever a person's background. Japanese people today may strike Westerners as proud or even precious about their company uniforms, as particular about their choice of tie, or even peculiar in their fashion choices outside work—such as taking part in anime conventions, where people may dress up as one of their favorite anime or computer game characters (a pastime known as costume-play or cosplay, now popular all over the world). But remember that all this passion for dressing up comes from a real enthusiasm for fashion and style, and a genuine feeling of pride in what they are wearing and what their clothes say about the way they live their lives.[23]

I think we can all learn from this arguably more democratic idea of fashion—not letting ourselves be told what to wear, but starting to think about our style from a place of respect: respect for ourselves and respect for what we do. There is creativity as well as discipline in tailoring what we wear to different parts of our lives, whatever we do for a living.

*Occasion—finding your balance with others* • Certain patterns, such as icy blue snowflakes or falling rain, are said to have a cooling effect on the people around you as they appreciate the iciness of the patterns. Giving others a small reminder of the changing seasons, or sharing feelings with others through the clothes we wear, is what kimonos are all about: a sense of coolness in the summer, a sense of the fleeting beauty of spring with cherry blossom motifs, or a sense of nostalgia in the patterns of falling leaves in the autumn.

This idea of dressing in harmony with others may strike some readers as alien. In the West, we often talk about making a fashion statement—when our clothes say something exciting and individual about us. *Chōwa* doesn't stamp out individual expression, but it does encourage us away from fashion "statements" and toward fashion "conversations." Thinking about what our clothes are saying also requires us to pay attention to what other people are wearing, just as dressing in harmony with nature requires us to pay close attention to the seasons. Showing off our sensitivity to the way others dress and what we are contributing to a wider, lively discussion is just as important for showcasing our creativity and flair as choosing the loudest outfit we own.

Thinking about what we wear through the lens of *chōwa* is not just a matter of fitting in. It's about being mindful of the impression we're creating, whatever we're wearing.

Forget the language of competition, rivalry, and intimidation that is drilled into us by fashion magazines and advertising. Try complimenting others on the clothes they're wearing and deliberately creating an atmosphere of happy, casual confidence with what you're wearing.

## Finding your style

While the kimono may be renowned for its timeless elegance, its intricate rules, and its special relationship with nature, Japanese fashion is also famous for its originality. Its patterns, cuts, and colors can be highly stylized—think Tokyo street fashion, like the hyper-cute *kawaii* style, which features shocking pinks, frills, and accessories decorated with anime and pop-culture characters—or minimal and stripped down, like the distressed kimono-inspired silhouettes by designer Yohji Yamamoto, cut from a single sheet of fabric.

Whatever designs or styles people are drawn to, I think that the originality in Japanese style comes from the clash between a culture of dressing by the book and efforts to break out. In Japan, it can seem like only the bravest and the most passionate people can find the courage, and the time, to be different. Daily life in Japan can be very strict and controlled. When I was young, it wasn't uncommon for teachers to go around the class with a ruler to check the length of girls' skirts. Even today, young people preparing for job interviews will all be required to cut their hair in the same way (this is known as the recruit cut) and even go out and purchase a specific kind of suit (known as the recruit suit).

Many of the young people I know in Japan are wary about expressing what makes them stand out. This fear of being unusual is particularly pronounced in Japan, but at times we all find it difficult to square what we believe to be our role in society with what we'd dearly love to express to others about ourselves.

In this final section of the chapter, I want to look at what *chōwa* can teach us about doing things in our own unique way. Having confidence in our personal style and learning to stand by what makes us different could help us find out who we really are. Then all we need to do is find the courage to share this with others.

*Root yourself by finding what you really love* • It may be hard to believe but, apart from a few replacements and repairs, I have rarely gone shopping for clothes over the last twenty-five years.

When I was first married, my husband's family took me to Paris. It was the first time I had been to Europe. The clothes in the Paris boutiques we visited took my breath away—the patterns, the textiles, and the colors were so alien to me. It was like looking at foreign works of art. I still own all the beautiful clothes I brought back with me from that trip. I find them just as beautiful today as I did then. Some people say that my taste in clothes is old-fashioned, but I happen to think that beautiful things remain beautiful.

My mother subscribed religiously to Japanese fashion magazines. Living on my grandmother's remote farm meant there was very little by way of entertainment for my mother, apart from a visit to the movies once a month. So she spent all her money from her part-time jobs—sewing kimonos and working in a hospital— on beautiful clothes. She would take a picture of a beautiful dress to the local tailor and say, "Make this for me, please." She is now in her eighties and no longer has the opportunity to wear them, so these clothes have been passed on to me. They include a classic, made-to-order navy woolen coat with a stripy grey-and-white collar and two suits—one black with a luxurious silk lining and one stunning dark purple suit. When I wear these sixty-year-old suits, tailor-made for my mother but which fit me almost perfectly, it feels a little like she's here with me.

One of my favorite kimonos once belonged to my grand-mother. It has a dragonfly on its back. The dragonfly is an important insect in martial arts as it is said to have a 360-degree field of vision. You can imagine why, for a warrior, having a wide field of vision—being able to see behind as well as in front—would be a valuable asset. Whenever I feel that I need to ready myself for an important event, one in which I have to be at my most alert, I wear this kimono. It helps me feel rooted and stable, a little like my grandmother is protecting me.

- Do you have certain items of clothing that carry a sense of history? Were they hand-me-downs from an older sibling, or clothes you bought from a vintage clothing shop that feel special to you? If you haven't worn them for a while, can you think of any ways to incorporate them back into the kind of outfits you wear every day? There's nothing like the sensation of wearing a piece of your own personal history to remember exactly who you are.

- Have you ever thought about which items of clothing make you happy? Ask yourself why they make you so happy. What is it about these items that make you feel excited to wear them, or more relaxed, or more yourself? Now try doing the same thing for clothes that don't make you happy. Ask yourself why you don't like wearing them. Are they too formal? Do you feel that they don't say what you want to say about yourself?

*Style is sharing what you love with others* • The last time my daughter and I went to Japan, my daughter bought a magazine to read on the train. It was called *Tsurutokame* ("the crane and the tortoise"). It's a fashion and lifestyle magazine aimed both at senior citizens and at the younger generation looking for inspiration from their quirky, retro fashion sense. The magazine was full of images of senior citizens, many of them rural workers, craftspeople, and street-food vendors. The text described them—the pride they took in their work or hobbies, as well as containing darkly comic sections about how much medication they had to take each day. A full-page picture showed an elderly gentleman winking as he looked over his shoulder, straddling his mobility scooter in a pose straight out of *Easy Rider*. There was a close-up of a woman's wrinkled face, her brow furrowed as she slurped her noodles, forgetting the photographer was even there at all. A woman grinning, baring her prominent gold tooth. What tied all of the pictures together was how happy and confident the models seemed. It wasn't just what they were wearing. No matter how unusual their hobbies, or their lifestyles, or poses—relaxing naked in a hot spring or scowling over a garden fence with a rock star attitude—they were so full of life. They all had style.[24]

In Japan, people have a great deal of respect for senior citizens, even if they can be rather eccentric. But I do worry sometimes whether this is at the expense of young people, who are expected to show no such eccentricities or quirks of their own. Young people are expected to get in line, follow the rules, and live the same regimented, orderly lives as the generation that preceded them. Some young people resist conformity and are proud of what makes them stand out. But many young people I know in Japan, who love counter-culture fashion, cosplay, or *kawaii* style, feel pressurized into conforming with an old-fashioned set of values—at least on the outside. Not wanting to embarrass their parents or get an earful from their elderly neighbors, they bundle their more daring clothes and accessories into a rucksack, sneak out and get an early train to the city, where they will change in a public restroom. I know that the young people aren't to blame here—they are only doing their best to manage the expectations of their community with their desire to do their own thing. Neither are their neighbors to blame. But I can't help thinking that all this secrecy and shame is a wasted opportunity.

Wouldn't it be wonderful if we could start to have more productive discussions with one another about what makes us tick, so that we can stop hiding and start sharing more? I can't see any other way toward lasting harmony unless we learn to share, and appreciate what other people are passionate about.

*Accepting what makes you different and leading with it* • No matter how much people love it when I wear a kimono in London, there is no denying that it calls me out as different. People might say, "What a unique outfit! Where are you from?" It is almost always positively meant, but it can be hard to take as a compliment. In Japan, the word *unique* has a strongly negative connotation: "her style is unique" has a pointed, slightly unpleasant meaning, i.e., "she's doing something *really* off the wall."

I came to accept my own unique style by asking myself what I really liked about wearing a kimono. Even though it meant looking different from other people in London, what was it about wearing a kimono that I couldn't give up?

What it came down to was a certain feeling. Wearing a kimono gives me the same feeling of uprightness and comfort in London as it gives me in Japan. It keeps my tummy in, my back straight. I feel like I can almost glide through the world. Wearing a kimono also makes me feel proud and happy to be Japanese. This can be useful, like when groups of lost Japanese tourists in Leicester Square come over to me as soon as they see what I'm wearing, and I'm usually able to help them find wherever they're going.

When we start to lead with what we feel makes us different from others—even with what we feel makes us unique—this can actually help us to find our tribe. This can be a great feeling, particularly when the people who find us are struggling with their own style, or feel literally, or metaphorically, lost.

We spend our lives living shoulder to shoulder with others. Pride. Confidence. Courage to accept who we are—these are all powerful values. When we lead with what makes us different, we send a powerful outward sign of inner commitment to others: that we will accept what makes other people different too.

*Don't just stand out—stick out all the way* • A common proverb in Japan is *deru kūi wa utareru* (the nail that sticks out gets
hammered down). It's written as:

> 出る杭は打たれる

This is often used to suggest that, in Japan, it is hard, or
somehow wrong, to stand out in any way. The smallest devia-
tion from the norm is met with resistance, even horror. There is
something violent about this image, isn't there, especially if we
imagine ourselves as the nail. It is hard to avoid the fact that,
in Japan, this proverb sometimes rings true. There is a certain
kind of person who takes pleasure in telling others what they
should do. If we are to change things for the better, particularly when it comes to the way society frowns on certain styles
or ways of living or loving, our best hope is not only to stick
out a little, but to stand out all the way so there is nothing
anyone can do about us. We need to shine.

Throughout my life, I have always done things my own
way—always stuck out a little, you might say—and quite often
I have been bullied and criticized for doing so. I was bullied
rather badly at school. Even when I left Japan for the UK, as
I continued to do things my own way, I was seen by some
members of the Japanese community in London as a difficult
woman, someone who did things her own unique way. In particular, setting up my charity led to the wrong kind of attention

from people who thought I should stick my neck out a little less. It hasn't always been easy.

I used to dream that I was back at school, being taunted by a bunch of bullies from my childhood. It was a recurring nightmare. I was upset when the dream came back again in my adulthood, just when I thought I was feeling settled in England, in my new life. Evidently I was still worrying about things subconsciously, things that made me different from those around me. I ended up telling my friend about it. She laughed.

"*Akemi san*, you are no longer *deru kūi* [the nail that sticks out]," she said. "You are *de sugi chatta* [the nail that sticks out *far* too much]!"

She told me that for as long as she'd known me, I'd always done my own thing. In the past, people had beaten me down and told me I couldn't do certain things—as a divorced woman, as the wife of a foreigner, or as a Japanese person.

My friend went on. "For better or worse, you're no longer the person you used to be. You've spent so long doing your own thing that there's no way anyone could beat you down. You're the nail that no one could hammer down even if they tried."

Here's another Japanese proverb that may be useful if you're thinking about finding your own style, doing your own thing, and expressing what makes you who you are:

継続は力なり
*Keizoku wa chikara nari*
"Persistence is power"

Strictly, this can be translated as "strength from continuation," but I prefer "persistence is power." If you care enough about something, the more you practice it—whether it's a hobby, a skill, a certain way of living, or a job—the better you will become at it. Eventually, it can become as natural as breathing. That is how we become who we want to be: we find what we love and we keep at it. When we know who we are, and what we truly care about, we feel less pressure to follow fashion, see the latest must-see movie, or keep up with the Joneses.

- Finding our style is as simple as learning how to live, work, dress, and move through the world with confidence, pride, and honor. The happier we are with ourselves, the more confidence we have, and the more ready we are to help other people.

## A day at the races

My daughter and I were once invited to attend the races at Royal Ascot. Nothing we owned seemed to fit with the dress code we were expected to follow. But, after debating what we would wear, I decided to wear a kimono, even if I wasn't sure this was strictly in line with the rules.

When we arrived, I felt quite lost in a sea of stately women. They all seemed to be competing over who had the largest, most outrageous hat. I also wore a hat, inspired by a twelfth-century-style veil that I thought was in keeping with my kimono and had the added benefit of hiding my face. (My daughter and I, finding something particularly amusing about some of the extraordinary outfits we saw, sometimes struggled to keep a straight face.)

We stood just outside the Royal Enclosure, an invitation-only space for people of a certain class, it seemed. All I could think, standing there in my light-blue kimono, was that I was going to be exposed as an outsider at any moment. Sipping champagne and eating strawberries, all the women wearing such beautiful dresses, I felt out of place.

After a while, a group of women came up to us. They were full of questions about my kimono, and I started to relax a little at last. I realized that, while I couldn't compete with their elegant style, I had brought my own style. I had honored my roots and still somehow managed to pass in the company of these people, for whom style was a serious matter. I feel that my kimono allowed me to fit in at the same time as it allowed me to stand out—that's the kind of balance I think we are often trying to strike when we are deciding what to wear. When we get it right, it can be a real thrill.

## Dressing in harmony with the seasons

*Winter colors*
Green with orange, red with white, or green with white

*Winter patterns*
Bamboo, pine, camellia, or *ume* (plum blossom)

*Spring colors*
Pink with white and green, purple with white, or light yellow with a darker yellow

*Spring patterns*
*Ume* (plum blossom) or *sakura* (cherry blossom)

*Summer colors*
Icy blue, lavender, or dark blue

*Summer patterns*
Rain and/or falling snowflakes, plain or striped *yukata*-style patterns (summer *yukata* are often navy on white or white on navy)

*Autumn colors*
Purples with oranges and greens or reds, oranges, and yellows (like falling leaves), or yellows and oranges (to capture the quality of autumn sunlight)

*Autumn patterns*
Falling leaves, sunlight through the trees, pampas grass, the moon or the dragonfly

## *Chōwa* lessons:
## finding your style

**Learn what you love, then share it with others**

- Find out what you care about.

- Put aside time each day to do it. And stick to it.

- Remember, "persistence is power."

- Now ask yourself, how can you share your passion with others?

**"The nail that sticks out gets hammered down"**

- What things make you feel like you stick out?

- How could you turn this difference on its head to embrace what makes you unique, so you can become "the nail that no one could hammer down, even if they tried"?

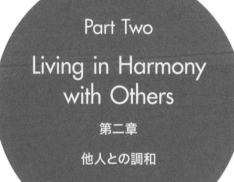

Part Two

Living in Harmony
with Others

第二章

他人との調和

# 5

## Listening to Others and Knowing Ourselves

*Saying nothing can be as beautiful as a flower.*
—Japanese proverb

We live with others. They keep us company, they support us, they guide us, and sometimes they can hurt us very badly. How we treat them, and how they treat us in return, is a large part of who we are. But while we spend every day of our lives in the company of others, we can often feel like we don't understand them very well. A misunderstanding or a harsh word can make us doubt our closeness to a friend, a colleague, or a partner, and upsets our own emotional balance. One of the most painful feelings is feeling that you have let someone down: emotions such as guilt, shame, or a sense of not being good enough can be persistent and overwhelming. If we let them, they can take over our lives.

As I've said, the Japanese word for self is *jibun*, which literally means "the self-part." This suggests that we are part of a larger whole. If we think about our greatest problems—feelings of insecurity, of not living up to expectations, heartbreak, anger, or failure—they usually relate to other people. Have you noticed that when a colleague or a family member is in a bad mood, their mood affects us? We have an emotional ecosystem that, just like the natural world, hangs in an often precarious balance. Finding our balance is not a question of bringing peace and harmony to our emotional lives. Emotions come and go. Our mental state is constantly changing. But what we can do is commit to spending our lives actively living in harmony with other people. This chapter introduces a few principles that might help you live a more healthy emotional life. The most important lesson is that our own personal balance begins by being more alert to the emotional lives of others.

- **Read the air.** A life lived in accordance with *chōwa* helps us to develop a high level of emotional sensitivity. By learning to tune in to the atmosphere of a room, into the here and now of a conversation, we learn how to observe our passing thoughts more calmly, and—in a more relaxed and receptive state—become better at setting others at ease.

- **Improve your relationships and learn how to handle intense emotions.** It can feel impossible to center ourselves when we are dealing with difficult emotions, such as anger and frustration. *Chōwa* can help us rethink our relationships with these powerful negative emotions and make our relationships with others easier to manage too.

I'd like to share with you a poem that my father wrote:

> When you look in the mirror, how do you see yourself?
> If you cannot see yourself clearly, maybe you are not happy.
> When your mind is cloudy, you cannot see yourself clearly.
> Even when you wipe the mirror, you cannot see yourself
> clearly.
> Do you appreciate everyday life?
> Do you work with honor?
> Do you help people who need your help?

The poem moves from thinking about oneself, from the recognition that you are not happy, to questions that encourage us to stop looking inward and to connect again with the wider world. When it comes to achieving personal balance, expanding our sphere of awareness to include others might sound counterintuitive, but I find it makes most sense to start here.

## Reading the air

Have you ever avoided a topic or chosen your words carefully so you don't make someone else feel uncomfortable? Have you ever closed a door quietly to prevent disturbing your child, or your partner, or a housemate when they have been hard at work or fast asleep? If so, you may already have learned to practice a technique Japanese schoolchildren are taught early in life. In Japanese, this skill is referred to as reading the air:

---

空気を読む

*kuuki wo yomu*

---

Reading the air is about being still and quiet so you can pick up on tiny shifts in the atmosphere, whether in a classroom, meeting, or family gathering. Think of it as taking the emotional temperature in a room. You can even practice it in one-on-one situations. It's not just about guessing how another person might feel; it's about active ways of creating peace, harmony, and quiet through very small actions. It takes a lifetime to develop, but it's a lot less mystical than it sounds. To do it, you have to tune in to what's going on with you, at the same time as tuning in to what's going on with someone else. I believe it can be taught in a few simple steps.

*Practice being quiet* • In Japan there is a saying: "quietness is the oil that makes everything run smoothly." The first trick in reading the air is to practice being quiet. This doesn't mean you switch off from what's going on. Think of yourself as a receiver, an instrument to pick up unspoken signals. When there is a pause in conversation, or an uncomfortable silence, you may feel that you should fill that silence. But talking isn't always as useful as we think.

*Let the other person go first* • All conversations are a search for balance. But sometimes we can treat our conversations with others more as competitions. When we are speaking to someone, it can be tempting to launch into our news or what we want to say before we've asked them anything. Letting the other person go first, and asking questions, will show them that you are really listening. This is known as active listening. You will be surprised by how quickly the other person will start to put you first too. The more we practice active listening, the more others will start to follow our example.

*Advice can wait* • Whether you are having a meeting about a problem at work or trying to listen to your child about a difficulty they are facing at school, I'm sure you will have had the impulse to advise, offer suggestions, or relate what is being said back to your own experience: "That's just like what's going on with me . . ." The "me, me, me" impulse does not necessarily come from a bad place. We want to show others that we empathize. But it can get in the way of true understanding. *Chōwa* requires us to do our research before we act to bring balance to a situation. When we are talking to another person, this means really listening to what is going on with them. Even if the other person has stopped talking, let what they have said sink in before you reply. Giving them a few more moments of silence also gives them space to say more, if they want to.

*Respond generously* • When you are listening to someone, particularly if they are telling you about something personal or painful, try asking yourself, "How can I make this person feel more comfortable?" Something very small, like a smile, or asking an open question, could set them at ease. Or, if you're comforting a close friend, try telling them that you understand, that you're listening, and that you're there for them. Create a moment of quiet so they can say more if they need to, or they can remain silent if they like.[25]

*Extend your emotional attention to include others as well as yourself* • Extending your emotional attention to include others is as simple as doing your emotional homework. This is about knowing what is going on with you and thinking a little more consciously about what is going on with other people.

When we replay a conversation in our head—as we often do if we feel we have put our foot in it—we realize that, if we have said something unhelpful, or even unpleasant, it was probably because we felt nervous, frustrated, angry, or keen to make someone else like us. We end up saying things to others that we regret when we allow ourselves to be governed by these emotions. We can avoid situations like this by trying to relate to our emotions with a little more level-headedness. The next time you feel overwhelmed, or swept up by an emotion, try silently telling yourself, "This is what anger feels like," or "This is what frustration feels like." Practice naming and identifying how you are feeling, particularly if you feel as if you might say something you'll regret. You'll notice, when you pay attention to how you feel in a softer, more objective way, your emotions start to have less of a hold on you.

Once you have stepped back from your thoughts and learned to observe them passing a little more objectively, you will be in a better place to focus on how other people are feeling. The next time you are speaking to someone, try extending your emotional attention to others as well as yourself. Try asking yourself, "How are they doing?" By starting to pay better attention to others, and what might be going on with them, we start to take a more active interest in our emotional ecosystem. We should always remember that we are all part of the same emotional ecosystem. Usually, if the balance in a room is off, so is our own personal balance. Consciously checking in, even if we don't do it aloud, with how others are doing, helps us respond more kindly. For example, if a colleague zones out in a meeting, you could ask them a direct question to bring them back into the fold. Or, if a friend is a little quieter than usual, try giving them an opening to talk about something you know they enjoy discussing. One generous act can breathe new energy into a room. And when one person starts to show a little more consideration to others, everyone will start to see the benefits of sharing the emotional load.

- What can you do to make small, positive impacts on your emotional ecosystem today?

- At the end of the day, ask yourself how things have gone, whether you have been trying to listen more actively or simply be more present with others in general. Did this allow you to calm a confrontation or help someone to feel more at ease in your company?

## Emotional check-ins

After my daughter was born, I was no longer responsible just for how I was feeling. I had to attune myself to her needs and emotions: Was she hungry? Was she tired? Was she too hot or too cold?

This attentiveness continued as she grew older. Whenever my daughter got home from school, I would stop what I was doing when I heard the door close. Was the door slammed? Or was it closed quietly? This was my first clue to how my daughter's day had gone and how she was feeling. Then I would hear her yell "*Tadaima!*" I'm back. I would say "*Okaerinasai.*" Welcome home.

If my daughter yelled "*Tadaima*" in a bright, breathless way, I imagined that she had been chatting with friends and had raced home so she wasn't late to help me with the cooking. But if she said "*Tadaima*" in a dull, sluggish way, I might worry that something bad had happened—that she had fallen out with a friend or received a bad grade.

You might have a similar call and response with members of your own family. Remember to take time each day to check in emotionally on your loved ones. If you do, you will be able to see when anyone is unhappy or out of balance, and you will be able to respond.

## Likes and dislikes

Our likes and dislikes help us to forge friendships and even to find romantic partners. We naturally gravitate toward people who are similar to us, who like the same things as we do—people we feel we have things in common with. But expressing strongly held preferences can sometimes get us into trouble.

In Japan, being overly attached to likes and dislikes is sometimes seen as childish or even selfish, something that makes us less able to be considerate of other people. For example, even when declining an invitation or permission or another piece of cake, Japanese people will be unlikely to say no. Rather than refuse explicitly, we say *chotto*, which means something like "it's a little bit difficult." Even when it comes to things we would really rather not do, or eat—perhaps we have an aversion to mushrooms or a certain kind of fruit—we will rarely outright refuse it, and we would be very unlikely to express a strong dislike. This may sound self-effacing or overly meek. Sometimes it can be exhausting, it's true, but at the same time, our dislikes can be like a series of locked doors that dictate how we live our lives: we have to avoid spending time with that person, avoid listening to that kind of music, avoid eating that kind of food. There can be a real relief when we free ourselves from the ideas we have held—often since childhood—about what we like and dislike. Being more flexible is not about compromising about who we are, but about keeping our options open and learning to go with the flow a little more. We may find that we are more flexible and adventurous than we may give ourselves credit for.

To illustrate how we can take a slightly more flexible approach toward our personal likes and dislikes, I'm going to give you a very basic lesson in Japanese grammar. Japanese grammar can be perplexing for students with English as their first language. The word order seems completely topsy-turvy—the verb comes at the end of the sentence. Also, pronouns are rarely used. Usually people understand by the context whether you are saying "Do you like apples?" or "I like apples."

Take, for example, the sentence "I like apples."

> 林檎　が　好き　です
> *ringo　ga　suki　desu*
> (I) Apples like do

*Ringo* means apples. *Ga* is a participle which, with *suki*, means "I like." But what makes this sentence mean "*I do* like apples" rather than "*I do not* like apples"? It's the word at the end, *desu*. "I do not like apples" would be:

> 林檎　が　好き　で　は　ありません
> *ringo　ga　suki　de　wa　arimasen*
> (I) Apples　like　do not

This makes listening to Japanese a real test of your attention. You have to wait until the end of a sentence to work out what the person is saying. But this also gives Japanese speakers time to think about what they are going to say. They can postpone coming down on either side—"Do I like apples, or do I not like apples?"—until the last moment.

If your host asks you, for example, "Do you like apples?" you might not want to express your dislike of apples straightaway. She may have made an apple pie for dessert.

Take a little extra time. This can prevent you from putting your foot in it or hurting another person's feelings when you express a personal preference.

Put personal preferences to one side. *Chōwa* is not about keeping silent about our preferences or opinions in the interest of social harmony. It's about keeping our options open, being mindful and careful of others, and welcoming the release that comes when we free ourselves from fixed ideas about what we like and dislike.

## Dealing with people we don't like

What does it feel like to dislike someone? If you are like me, as you think about the negative feelings you have for another person, you might feel dislike and hatred entering your body like a kind of pain. Your face may feel rigid or you may feel a tension in your jaw and the back of your neck.

Don't feel bad, we've all been there. But if you take a moment to reflect on these feelings, you may realize you don't have to feel this way.

When I was newly married, I attended the same tea ceremony class as a woman named Akiko. She, like me, was a newlywed. Unlike me, she had a cruel wit and an unpleasant sense of humor. She delighted in teasing others in the class, lauding her status as a newly married woman and taking pot shots at anyone who made a mistake. I found it almost impossible to be in the same room with her. At one point my frustration boiled over. I blew out my cheeks and sighed loudly. When Akiko looked up, I hid my sour expression, pretending to be very interested in my fan.

My mother-in-law, who attended the class with me, had noticed. As we were returning home, she asked, "What is it with you and Akiko-san?"

"I don't know. I just don't like her," I said honestly. There were too many reasons.

"Is there anything you do like about her?" asked my mother-in-law, kindly.

I considered her question. I did like Akiko's naughty sense of humor. And when I really thought about it, some of the things I disliked about Akiko were things I worried about myself: was I becoming more stuck up, worrying too much about pleasing people or about being caught doing the wrong thing?

*Chōwa*, as well as teaching us how to change our attitudes toward our preferences, can teach us how to transform our attitudes toward other people. Giving ourselves the opportunity to change a relationship with someone we find difficult, or dislike, can be a huge weight off our shoulders.

## Dealing with difficult emotions

I try to take a philosophical approach to difficult emotions. When I'm angry, sad, frustrated, or in any kind of physical pain, I try to tell myself, this is life. You are living. When bad things happen, my bad feeling is a natural, emotional response to them. Even if it really hurts, these feelings are part of life and there is something beautiful about them. But in the midst of a rage, or in the depths of shame, thinking like this is much easier said than done.

Here are a few ideas for dealing with two of the most painful emotions. The first is often directed at other people: anger. The second is usually directed at ourselves: frustration.

*Anger* • There are times when anger does us no good at all, as I am sure we all know too well. Anger blinds us to our own faults. It makes it harder for us to put ourselves in other people's shoes. Responding to a situation with anger can turn into a bad habit, whether it's overreacting to someone who has bumped into us on the street or when a friend has made an honest mistake.

On one hand, our anger makes sense. We want to tell someone off, to make someone else understand how we feel. But you could try communicating how you feel in a different way.

Try responding in the opposite way. If someone shoves you on a bus, try laughing rather than snapping at them. If someone says something you fiercely disagree with, try telling them, "I can see that's how you feel about it." It's as much about disarming your own anger as it is about disarming the other person, particularly if they are looking for an argument. Bringing balance to such encounters can make it more pleasant for us all to move through the world, and allows people who are just looking for a fight to go quietly on their way.

## Write down your "righteous" anger

I once received a call from my friend Junko-san. We had a lot to catch up on, but eventually our conversation turned to her fiancé. They had had a big argument. The argument had ended with him shouting at her at the top of his lungs. I was surprised that she sounded so calm, almost cheerful, about it.

She told me that during the argument she had walked away into another room, leaving her fiancé standing there, fuming. She quietly closed the door of the dining room. She took three deep breaths. She let her heart rate slow down. She sat down at the dining table with a piece of paper. She wrote down everything she was feeling in the form of a letter to her fiancé. It articulated why she felt that his shouting at her was unacceptable, however angry he was. She wrote that she wasn't prepared to enter a marriage where this kind of shouting was going to be a part of their everyday lives. When she had finished writing all of this down, she came back and handed him the letter. At first, he was even angrier. She explained that she had been too angry to say what she was feeling, so she had written it down instead.

She told him that he was free to do the same, then left the house to play tennis with her friends. When she returned home, she found a written apology from her fiancé lying on her dressing table.

Examine your anger so it can work for you, not against you. I have heard of other Japanese women using Junko-san's technique: writing their anger on a piece of paper and handing it to their husband. The next time you get angry with your spouse, or your roommate, try it.

*Frustration* • The search for balance is not always an easy one. You will encounter setbacks, obstacles, and times when you feel stuck. Frustration is one of the most painful human emotions. We expect so much of ourselves and we can be our own worst critic. Sometimes our expectations are too high, and we end up disappointed. This is a well-known proverb in Japanese:

七転び八起き
*nana korobi yaoki*

It means "if at first you don't succeed, try, try again." To me, this proverb captures how we feel when we don't succeed better than the English version, because it is literally translated as: "Fall down seven times, get up eight times." We all need to accept that we are going to fall, more than once. My advice is to make peace with it, and keep going. You will fall seven times. You might even fall more than seven times. What is important is that you pick yourself back up again.

## Some problems are too big to fix

My first husband and I divorced in 1989. Even while I knew it was the right thing to do, I had very little idea what I was going to do next. After my divorce, I started to realize that it was not something in me that was out of balance. It was my environment, the whole world around me, that was broken. I felt as if I could see the society in which I lived clearly for the very first time.

The divorce meant that I had to find a job to support myself and my baby daughter. But so much of the work I was interested in required me to declare my marital status. Writing "divorced" on job application forms closed a great number of doors to me. I also had to find a nursery school for my daughter—but even here I was asked why I was a single mother. Being a divorced parent was almost unheard of in Japan at the time. The more I thought about it, the less I wanted my daughter to be brought up in a society like this. I was worried that, if we stayed in Japan, my daughter and I would keep being knocked down like this, again and again, until we were destroyed.

Sometimes, we blame ourselves for problems that have really nothing to do with us, such as a toxic workplace or a bullying partner.

In these situations, try as we might to bring a little balance to our environment, we can rarely change other people. It is almost impossible to improve an environment that is simply not good for us. So sometimes the only thing to do, the best thing for us, as painful as it may be, is to make a clean break and move on.

## *Chōwa* lessons:
### listening to others and knowing ourselves

**Listening to others**

Try to practice listening more actively by:

- Being quiet (really paying attention to what the other person is saying).

- Letting the other person go first (let them share their news before you share yours).

- Waiting. Sometimes silence is the best response; the other person may have more to say.

- Doing what you can to respond generously, whether that involves saying something or nothing at all. Ask yourself, how can I make this person feel more comfortable?

### Dealing with people you don't like

- Think of someone you don't like. List the things you don't like about them.

- Now try to list the things you do like about them.

- Keep going until the list of things you do like is at least as long as the list of things you don't.

### Knowing yourself

Try asking yourself these questions, which were inspired by my father's poem:

- How can I better appreciate everyday life?

- How can I work with honor?

- How can I help other people?

6

# Learning to Learn, and Teaching Our Teachers

> "Hardships when we are young are good for us, even if we have to seek them out."
>
> —Japanese proverb

From the twelfth century to the 1870s, powerful *daimyo* lords ruled over much of Japan. Their warriors, the samurai, fought on their behalf for power and influence. Samurai were expected to learn a wide variety of warrior arts including *iaidō* (the art of drawing one's sword), *battōdō* (the art of using one's sword), and *bushidō* (the warrior code of ethics). But after the battle was over, samurai would return to their families. They mostly led peaceful lives, living off the land. Just as important to a samurai's education were artistic pursuits such as *shodō* (the art of calligraphy), *kadō* (the art of flower arrangement), and *chadō* (the art of tea), as well as learning how to run a farm. It was a balanced education, informed not by conflict but by how to live in harmony with one's family and appreciate the beauty of the natural world during peace time.

Modern Japanese education places a similar emphasis on "all-rounders." Rather than focusing solely on academic work, a Japanese education teaches children the value of teamwork, how to get along well with others, and how to develop into a thoughtful person who is good at reading the air, whether in the classroom or the workplace. I have lived and taught in the UK and in Japan. I have seen firsthand that a Japanese education can focus a little too much on learning to fit in. It seems to me that at all stages in life, we need to learn to accommodate the needs of the group and to question the principles of harmony that hold that group together. Here are the key lessons this chapter will discuss.

- **Learn how to learn.** *Chōwa* is about being prepared to respond to any situation as bravely and positively as we can. I want to share how, when we infuse the way we learn with this idea, we not only learn more effectively but also carry on learning throughout our lives.

- **Teach your teachers.** The reluctance of students in Japan to voice their own opinions is well known in the West. But learning the right lessons from *chōwa* about actively seeking balance sometimes requires us to challenge authority, to challenge other people's ideas of what harmony means, to teach our teachers.

## Back to school—*chōwa* lessons in learning from a Japanese classroom

There is a great deal about English education that I really admire. I have visited all sorts of schools across the UK as both a Japanese teacher and a lecturer in cultural studies, and I have worked as a researcher for a Japanese broadcaster looking into what makes English education special. But there is nothing quite like stepping into a Japanese school to make one feel inspired and filled with an enthusiasm for learning. It is something I miss about Japan.

When people imagine a Japanese school, they might imagine that the teachers are very strict. There is some truth in this but, having visited all kinds of schools, in the West and in Japan, I can safely say that *chōwa* in Japanese classrooms is not about creating a group of identical students with the same opinions, learning together in a scary kind of harmony. In this chapter I will take you inside a Japanese classroom and share a few *chōwa* lessons with you to help guide you in your own lifelong education.

*Commit to your learning* • When you enter a Japanese elementary school, like entering a Japanese house, you step up into the corridor and take off your outdoor shoes. Students often have their own shoebox, but don't worry, there are indoor slippers for guests too. Changing our shoes before we step into the school is a small but simple way of making a distinction between the space in which we learn and the world outside. The first step to finding our balance in education is knowing that what we need when we study may not be what we need when we are not studying.

When you step into a Japanese classroom, many things may seem familiar. There's a whiteboard, rows of desks and chairs, boards for displaying students' work, and lockers for storing their bags. But as soon as a lesson begins, things might start to seem a little different.

Children are required to greet their teachers formally before the start of the lesson. When the teacher walks into the room, they might take some time to arrange their papers and wait for the children to quiet down. Then one member of the school group, the class leader, will lead the formal greeting to the teacher, saying in a firm voice:

> *Kiritsu*—stand up
>
> *Rei*—bow
>
> *Chakuseki*—take your seats

In other chapters we have spoken about the importance to *chōwa* of outward signs of inner commitment—making sure that our words are in harmony with our deeds. In a learning environment, these spoken commitments create a very particular kind of harmony. There is something powerful at the start of each lesson when all students are doing the same thing, consciously readying themselves to learn.[26]

**Make time to learn.** After we leave formal education, we have to motivate ourselves to keep learning, particularly if we are fitting in learning in our spare time or after work. Try making your learning environment different from your everyday environment, whether this means going to work in the local library or making a dedicated work space in your room. Keep blocks of time dedicated to learning. Set an alarm and put aside a good amount of time to work.

*Take care of your learning environment* • As soon as you step into a Japanese school building you will notice two things: the quiet atmosphere and how clean it is. Japanese students clean the school to show their gratitude for the service each space gives them: to thank the building, and their classrooms, for keeping them safe and giving them a space to learn.

Students are not only responsible for cleaning their own classrooms but also for cleaning the teacher's room, the corridors, and even the bathrooms and the school garden. Students do each job on a rotation, which gives them a sense of belonging not just to their class, but to the school.

As well as caring for the building, there is a deep sense of responsibility for the natural environment woven into a Japanese education. I recently took a group from a London primary school to visit a school in Tokyo. When we arrived, many of the children were out in the garden, pulling up weeds and planting seeds. One of the children from my group asked if it was some kind of punishment or detention. The headmaster, who was showing us around, shook his head. The students had volunteered to do this job in their break time—they found it fun and a way of giving back to the school.

*Match different kinds of learning with different kinds of teaching* • During my career as an educator, I have seen firsthand Japan's problems with teenage burnout, high school dropouts, and an overemphasis (from employers as well as educators) on pupils getting the best grades. Today, in the West, a Japanese education is often associated with high levels of competition and stress, as well as a rigid kind of uniformity in classroom etiquette.

What I do see sometimes in the UK, however, is the danger of rejecting methods of teaching that are not inherently bad. Take, for example, learning by rote, which seems to fill students in the UK, and their parents, with horror. It seems somehow Victorian to spend hours memorizing things by heart, or with one's nose pressed to a book. But as a language teacher I have to say that, as well as practicing speaking skills, learning a language requires dedicating a lot of time to some quite boring tasks, such as learning verb tables, vocabulary lists, and grammar rules. Like it or not, some subjects do involve learning by rote.

On the other hand, whether we are practicing a sport, complex forms of algebra, or trying to understand poetry, then merely learning the rules, the facts, or the words by heart is not likely to be the best way to learn. We have to learn by doing. We also need to know when to let ourselves be guided by intuition, by our hunches. The logic of a game, or an equation, or reading a novel, can take time to appreciate. We may need to give ourselves time to train, to learn, to read, and to think outside the box. Giving ourselves plenty of breaks is important for this kind of thinking.

As adults, we can be afraid to leave a book half finished and instead start another that has piqued our interest. Sometimes we need to allow ourselves to relax into our learning. Sometimes we need to reflect, to take stock of what we have learned. Sometimes, allowing our minds to wander can even lead to moments of inspiration.

There is no one right way to learn. We need to remember that different kinds of learning require different kinds of teaching.

*Success is not down to us alone* • When they are a little older, students and their parents will start to visit shrines before important exams to pray for a good result. Visiting a shrine is a physical, active reminder of how much we value our education—an outward sign of inner commitment. Going to a shrine or buying a good luck charm—while these things do need to be supported by actually studying—reminds ourselves and our families of our intentions and our values.

If we are lucky enough to get the grades we hope for, we will return to the shrine to say thank you. It's not just about saying thank you to the *kami*. It is a way of showing our gratitude more generally: to our parents, who supported us; to our teachers, who shared their knowledge with us; and to our friends, who helped us study (trips to the shrine are often made with one's classmates). You don't have to be religious to give thanks. An education infused with the ideas of *chōwa* teaches us that there is an equilibrium to learning; that it's not just about what we learn but who has taught us. We don't succeed on our own.

## Learn a language (to discover new kinds of balance)

When we are trying to find our balance, looking for the tools to learn and grow, learning a language can help us find the answer. Our own country's sense of *chōwa*—our national definition of what *harmony* means—can blind us to lessons we could learn from other countries. This is why, when it comes to finding your balance, learning a language is not only a life skill in itself, but it's also a doorway to knowledge that we never knew existed.

I have always been fascinated by the world outside Japan. When I was a child, American TV was very unlike much of Japanese entertainment at the time. It showed me that women could be both powerful and beautiful. When I watched shows like *Charlie's Angels* and *Bewitched*, I wondered how it might feel to be a free citizen of the world, and what mastering another language might offer me.

Let me share a few tips, both as a student and a teacher of languages.

*Work with what you know* • *Chōwa* teaches us to take the sum of our experience and our knowledge to make the best of any given situation. It is about harnessing what you know and not worrying too much about what you don't. In a new language, everything you learn—what you do know—becomes another exciting step to reaching the things you don't know yet. Being able to speak a few words in a new language will get you a long way. Here are some simple sentences in Japanese.

> *Watashi wa Akemi desu*—My name is Akemi
>
> *Hajimemashite*—How do you do?
>
> *Yoroshiku onegai shimasu*—It's nice to meet you

*Learn to think differently* • Learning a language can give us new tools to find our balance. Even learning a few words in another language can transform our thinking.

Take, for example, the Japanese for "it's nice to meet you." This is a very rough translation of what *yoroshiku onegai shimasu* means. It actually means something more like "thank you for taking so much trouble over me." You might say it when you meet someone for the first time. But you also might say it when you drop your child off at school, where it might mean "sorry that my daughter is such a handful." It's all about showing your humility and thanking others for taking care of you.

*Chōwa* informs a great deal of how the Japanese language is put together. Many of my students say they feel like it is a kind of antidote to the sort of thinking that prevails in English. I'm not immune to this either. I am always saying: "I'm so happy that . . ." or "I hope that . . ." There is a lot of "me, me, me" in English, and a lot of focus on how you are feeling. There is significantly less in Japanese.

In adapting to new ways of thinking when we learn a new language, we start learning to challenge our preconceptions of what it is to live and speak with other people, and what harmony really means.

*Be cautious about praise* • If you ever visit Japan and try speaking Japanese, you might hear the words "*nihongo ga jouzu desu ne.*" This means "your Japanese is very good." You should be rightly suspicious! While people are only trying to be polite, and it's unlikely they are making fun of you, the odds are that you still have a long way to go. I usually advise my students to reply with the phrase "*mada mada desu,*" which means "I still have a long way to go." It usually gets a laugh!

> まだまだ です
> *mada mada desu*

When you start what I have called the search for balance, we commit ourselves, just as we do when learning a language, to a lifelong process of learning. And like a language, it takes a lifetime to master.

## Lifelong learning: learning by doing

Before attending university in Saitama, I attended a finishing school where I studied Western etiquette. This might seem strange to readers who grew up in the West, who might think that etiquette lessons seem like something from the 1880s rather than the 1980s. But for me, this interest was perfectly natural. When I was young, I was captivated by Western culture. I wanted to learn more about the rules and codes that lay behind the elegant surface of these people's daily lives.

Learning how to walk like a Western woman was, literally, its own lesson in finding my balance. I had to learn to sit and stand with a book on my head, keeping my posture straight. I learned how to walk in Western clothes and Western shoes. In a kimono, one takes small steps. When one is wearing a dress and high heels, one has to stride with more confidence. At first it certainly wasn't a natural way of holding myself.

*Never stop learning* • Some of us consider, when we leave school or university, that our education is over. Not so in Japan. *Chōwa* encourages us to keep learning, moment by moment, and to see education as something that continues all our lives, whether you're getting to grips with new technology at work or teaching yourself a new skill like playing a musical instrument or learning a language.

Even in retirement, senior citizens in Japan often end up taking leadership roles in their local communities: continuing their education is seen as both an enjoyable way to spend their time and a duty. Japan has one of the best education systems available to the elderly in the world.[27] After my mother retired, she decided to enroll in a horticulture course at university. She always liked working in the garden. Today, she is on her way to becoming a fully fledged horticulturalist. She often takes care of her neighbors' gardens for free.

Lifelong learning helps us prepare for anything. Some of my friends in the UK and Japan have experienced the shock of losing their job, or have reached retirement age without knowing what to do next. They have been really encouraged by my mother's example. Remember, the more you learn, the more prepared you are for the next stage in your life. Whatever we can bring to our situation, whatever we have learned, will be there to help us out in our most desperate hour.

As my grandmother used to say, "People can steal your jewels but they can't steal your education."

## Learning how not to fit in

At school, I had always enjoyed the company of boys my own age, so it was quite a shock when I ended up attending a girls' school in Saitama. I found the whole experience eerie. It was as if, without boys around, the girls had developed their own strange customs, such as hoisting up their skirts and using them to fan each other on hot days. They always insisted on going to the bathroom together, which I found very uncouth. When one girl asked me to go to the bathroom with her, I refused. I said, "What, can't you do it on your own?" She was fifteen years old. Clearly she didn't require any help in that department. She turned bright red and marched away. I felt that I'd held my own, but the other girls weren't impressed.

It was clear that I wasn't going to play their games. I wasn't going to fit in.

Looking back, all sorts of things happened at that school that I knew were quite ridiculous. But many people, wherever we live in the world, never grow out of the need to fit in, although perhaps this is more apparent in Japan than it is in England. When I travel back to Japan, I look around on the Tokyo Metro and see every woman my age clutching the same Louis Vuitton bag. There's no getting away from it. This is the price we pay for an education that emphasizes the importance of fitting in. It's one thing being able to adjust to adhere to the rules of an institution, doing what we can to make others feel comfortable and at ease; it's quite another to be afraid to do anything to show who we are.

I think this interpretation of *chōwa* is a gross misunderstanding of what it really means to search for balance. I believe that when it comes to finding our balance, we have to learn to stand up for what's important to us. At school, this took me some time to learn. But slowly I managed to find more productive ways of doing things my own way than making fun of the other girls, who, of course, had their own reasons for wanting to fit in. I joined the guitar and mandolin clubs, which allowed me to enjoy the company of like-minded girls. At the end of term, a group of boys from a school in Tokyo would come and watch us give a concert, so I also managed to make some friends outside school. We got teased for this, but we thought it was probably worth it.

## Teaching our teachers: arguing our way to harmony

A Japanese education can sometimes place too much emphasiz on group harmony, the kind of *chōwa* that can only be achieved by keeping one's head down and keeping quiet. We are told "don't talk back" and "don't argue" often enough that we give up. Learning how to question the way something is being done is a huge part of what an education should be about. It is also what *chōwa* should be about: the only way I know to seek balance is to develop the strength to see what is going on around us, to do our research, but also to challenge the status quo.

Here are some ways you can learn to argue your way to a better world with grace, but with persistence.

*Learning to argue—lessons from my students* • I don't think I knew the meaning of the words *argumentative* or *opinionated* until I taught British teenagers. Today, I still work as a teacher of Japanese in the UK. While my students are optimistic, eager, and bright, they are also individualistic and opinionated. I love it! They have helped me appreciate the value of putting your opinions out there, saying your piece, but at the same time being prepared to stand corrected and have your opinion scrutinized by others.

*Learning to argue—lessons from philosophy* • I have great respect for the Socratic method: that is, persistent, curious questioning, a relentless pursuit of the truth by asking, and asking, and asking again. This is not the "why, why, why" questioning of a child—a good question has to be supported by genuine interest; we are not simply trying to provoke a reaction. Socrates may have said that this can get us closer to the truth. I think we can also use this approach to bring us closer to balance.

Socrates' method was also good for exposing people who thought they knew it all. If someone said, "I think this is the truth," Socrates would ask, "But what about this?" It allowed the person, the questioner, and everyone listening to reassess, as well as generally encouraging an atmosphere of care and humility.

Never stop asking questions. When we ask questions with the right attitude, we can not only learn a lot more, but also, by encouraging our teachers to answer difficult questions, teach them a few things too.

## Learning the rules by breaking the rules

When I lived in Japan as a divorced woman, I realized quickly that I would be breaking the rules with every step of my new life. I had to learn how I was going to get away with this while keeping my sense of dignity and, of course, managing my career as a teacher.

When I got married for the second time, divorce was still a taboo topic in Japan. Worse still, I was getting married to a foreigner, to the English teacher who had become my business partner at my school. When we first went to the town hall, the officials refused to marry us—they had never married a Japanese woman to a foreigner before. We had to get the British embassy on the phone before they gave us our marriage certificate. I should have known then that staying in Japan was going to prove too difficult for both of us. Setback after setback encouraged us to move to England to start a new life there.

My experience of breaking the rules in Japan taught me a great deal about my country. The most important lesson I learned is that learning to question, to search for answers throughout our lives, is the only way we can ever hope to find our balance.

# *Chōwa* lessons:
# learning to learn

### Each subject is a search for balance

- What are you currently trying to learn or to get better at?

- What are your learning goals?

- How are you currently teaching yourself the new skill? Is this method helping you achieve your goal?

- Would trying a different learning style—either short bursts of cramming or longer periods of reflection—help you achieve your learning goals better?

### Learning to teach your teachers

Here is some inspiration for asking wiser questions of your teachers:

- Closed questions (those to which you reply yes or no) are not usually the most helpful, as they lead to no discussion.

- Always ask questions in good faith. Asking questions to which you already know the answer can sound confrontational.

- If you need something clarified, rather than asking an open question, try asking specific questions, "Please explain how . . ."

- Avoid "why, why, why" complaints disguised as questions. If you think something needs to be changed, be as specific as you can, do your research, or even suggest an alternative: "How about we try . . . ?"

- Prepare yourself for unexpected answers. A monk once asked his apprentice to clean the garden. The apprentice raked up all the leaves so that the garden was completely spotless. When the monk returned, the apprentice noticed that his teacher looked displeased.

   "Isn't the garden clean enough?" he asked his teacher.

   The monk shook a tree and a few leaves fell to the ground. "Now it is perfect," he said.

A mantra for learning, for teaching, and for life

- *Mada mada desu*—"I still have a long way to go."

# 7

# Bringing Balance to the Way We Work

> "Cultivate the right 'stance of mind.'"
> —Instruction for students of martial arts

The way we work is changing fast. We are more connected, doing business in multiple languages, across cultures, even across continents. Among my students, there is a real appetite for learning about *chōwa* and, in a business context, learning how to forge harmonious partnerships across cultures. (I run Japanese business etiquette classes in London, and I've never had more students.) But we are also seeing new fault lines opening up. Businesses the world over are being held to account for their greed, their lack of heart, their lack of values. We are learning, often too late, about the devastating effects of stress, bullying, and sex-based discrimination and sexual harassment in workplaces. This is just as true for the growing number of self-employed people who, especially when it comes to work-life balance, can be their own worst enemy. Recognizing these problems where they exist, while an important step, has not been enough to bring balance to the way we work.

I want to look at how *chōwa* can help us rethink the way we work. By approaching the way we work with the right "stance of mind," we can bring kindness and readiness to our work. We can also bring lessons we discussed in previous chapters—including learning how to listen more actively—to the way we work. They will teach us how to get along better with colleagues and clients, how to manage our work-life balance, how to voice disagreement constructively and question workplace harmony when it isn't working for us. This chapter will include these key lessons:

- **Be ready for anything.** I encourage you to approach work with the right mental stance, to remember "outward signs of inner commitment." Showing your commitment to your work can have a transformative effect on your workplace.

- **Remember your humanity.** Thinking about our work as a search for balance can allow us to appreciate how our workplaces function. We come to understand that companies, like any group of people, are always in a somewhat precarious harmony. We should not believe that workplace harmony is more important than telling the truth about abuse and overwork. We need to remind business leaders that some of us have put up with toxic working environments for far too long.

## Becoming a better person

A few years ago, I was invited to attend the World Martial Arts Festival in Kyoto. I was lucky enough to sit at the head table. Not only was I sitting at the table with some of Japan's top martial artists, but I was also sitting next to some of Japan's titans of industry. It was hard to tell them apart. In fact, many of Japan's top martial artists are also some of Japan's top business leaders.

Being in their company made me feel like I had to be on my best behavior. They all had such impeccable posture. I felt that I had to make a conscious effort to better my posture to match their example. Even the way they ate was skillful and confident. It was like watching people dance. At the same time, they were so relaxed and friendly.

The man on my left introduced himself as a judo practitioner. He turned out to be the CEO of a large software company. I asked him what had drawn him to martial arts. How could he do his job while keeping up this time-consuming and physically demanding hobby? His answer was simple. With a shrug and a smile he said, "I wanted to be a better person." He told me he had just been defeated in a judo match by a young Olympic hopeful. We started talking about judo as an Olympic sport. The CEO told me that he had mixed feelings about it. He really didn't see judo as a sport, but as an art. Gold, silver, and bronze medals didn't come into it. Before a match, one traditionally bows to a shrine in the dojo. If teachers are present, combatants will bow to their teachers. There is a sense of stillness and respect, along with an understanding that combat is a matter of life and death.

Of course, business thrives on competition but we cannot allow ourselves to forget how important our attitudes, values, and personality are to how we work. If a company, or an employee, has a reputation for sincerity, friendliness, and inner strength, then small losses and missteps can be dealt with gracefully: respect for our competitors. Preparation for our fights. Grace in our defeats. As in martial arts, these values allow us to handle even the most disappointing of outcomes. But when we are constantly striving to win, we can make ill-informed decisions, or fail to treat our colleagues with the respect they deserve, and we can forget how serious this is.

Perhaps, like judo, business is more of an art than a sport.

## *Kokoro gamae*: the right stance of mind

The *chō* of *chōwa* is a character that can be read as "search" and "study," but also as "preparation." I want to introduce you to a word in Japanese that has close ties to this reading of the *chō* character and can teach us a lot about the kind of readiness we need to find our balance at work. Even if this word is more usually associated with martial arts practice, it applies just as well to doing business with the right attitude:

---

心 構え

*kokoro gamae*

*Kokoro* literally means heart, but can also mean spirit or mind.

*Gamae* means posture or stance. As a verb, it means "to prepare."

---

The two characters combine to mean "state of mind" or even a "stance of mind." This is often translated into English as "readiness." In martial arts, *kokoro-gamae*—"readiness of the mind"—is linked closely to *mi-gamae*—readiness of the body (i.e., our physical stance, our readiness for a battle). This martial-arts-style readiness, in Japan, extends to the business world too. I think most of us would agree that if someone sits with their feet on their desk or acts like they don't care about their work, colleagues and clients are more likely to assume that they are not up to the job.

I can't tell you what readiness means in every job—it will mean something very different for a teacher than for a sales executive, for an architect than for a care worker. But I do want to explain what treating our business lives as a search for balance can do to bring stillness and kindness, energy and enthusiasm to our working lives, particularly when it comes to doing business with other people and building "harmonious partnerships" with clients.[28]

*Show you care* • Some Westerners think there's a stiff formality in the way Japanese people extend their arms, hand over their business cards with both hands and bow. But what can seem fussy to Westerners has real purpose and meaning.

How someone treats their business card is seen as a demonstration of their readiness, of their stance of mind. Being proud of your business card shows you are proud of your role in your company. The quality and condition of your business card (that it hasn't been crumpled in your pocket but kept in a special case) shows people how you will conduct business and how you are likely to conduct yourself.

When you receive someone else's business card, you are expected to spend several seconds looking carefully at the card, holding it by the corners so as not to obscure any information. Again, this is not just a formality. It shows that we value the person and their company.

*Don't be afraid of silence* • It is not uncommon for silence to fall in a meeting in Japan. Some of my British students find this unnerving. Have they said something terrible? Have they been offensive? The answer is usually no. Their counterparts in Japan are simply being polite, giving them a chance to speak if they would like to say more.

In Japan, it is said that silence is the oil that makes everything run smoothly. People expect there to be silence in business meetings in Japan because they expect everyone to be practicing active listening and reading the air. And as I mentioned earlier in the context of personal relationships, the same is true for our relationships with colleagues and clients. By paying attention to the atmosphere, we can learn a lot about the other people in it.

There are many benefits to a *chōwa*-style meeting where everyone is practicing reading the air and where we see quiet as allowing us to practice searching for balance as part of the meeting itself. Even if bringing more silence to a meeting is something you commit to on your own, you will find that your efforts are surprisingly contagious.

*Be patient* • As anyone who has ever done business in Japan will know, Japanese professionals need time to get to know you. The first meeting with a Japanese client is likely to be quite formal. So will the second and the third. But after this getting-to-know-you period, if you do end up doing business with Japanese clients, they can be some of the world's most loyal business partners. They can end up being far more than clients; they may end up becoming lifelong friends. I think this can apply to any client or colleague we have really taken the time to get to know properly.

So often in our professional lives, particularly if we are trying to sell ourselves, our company, or our company's services, we can end up forgetting the simple virtue of patience. We can end up exhausting ourselves by frantically trying to find things we have in common. A persistent approach can end up sounding desperate and needy: "Please like me, please like me!"

Most people we work with, in Japan or anywhere in the world, don't set out to like or dislike you. Instead, they want to learn more about your qualities, what you are like, and what it is like to do business with you. This takes time.

## Workplace *chōwa*—finding your balance at work

Finding your balance at work is rarely as simple as getting along well with your colleagues and clients. Expectations, deadlines, and tasks can stack up; we can find it difficult to manage the time we spend at work, to delegate tasks, or to make sure we come home on time, giving us enough time to live outside work.

Workplace *chōwa* is about paying attention to what is going on with other people, as well as what is going on with us. It also means knowing how to argue and state our case fairly, but with the courage of our convictions.

*Warming up before you start your day* • First thing in the morning, whether they work as cleaners, post-office workers, or in a large corporation, many employees in Japan do some light exercise while listening to calisthenics being broadcast on Japan's public radio service, NHK. It is quite a sight to watch groups of serious-looking company employees all moving in unison. These daily calisthenics are called *rajiotaisō*.

These light stretches get the blood moving and give staff a chance, from the CEO to the newest recruit, to move together and warm up for the day ahead.[29] Exercising on your own is a fine way to prepare for the day ahead, but exercising with colleagues can be an even better way of reminding everyone in the organization of some very obvious facts: that we are all the same and the success of our work depends on each and every one of us.

If you are going to try some communal exercise (even if it is just some light stretching) with your coworkers, I suggest starting with a couple of short sessions. Make sure you are mindful of other people's preferences, boundaries, and how much exercise they are comfortable doing.

*Be there for the people you work with: the* sempai/kōhai *mentor relationship* • Thinking about actively bringing balance to our lives does not stop when we leave the house in the morning. I find it sad that so many people stop thinking about others when they are working. Whether it's our clients or colleagues, or—in a more academic context like in my own work—students and teachers, we can gain a great deal from taking the time to engage with the people we work with.

In Japan, relationships between seniors and juniors are a little more formal—at least from my experience working with businesspeople in the West. We even refer to people who have just started at a company as *kōhai* (junior*)* and those above us as *sempai* (senior). I think spelling out these relationships a little more clearly has the benefit of emphasizing the *chōwa* lessons we learned in the previous chapter when it comes to teachers and students: in teaching relationships, respect isn't always a given; it's a balance we have to strike. While there may be a little teasing of one's *kōhai*, and while one has to address one's *sempai* with respect, the relationship is one of active mentoring and active learning. The *kōhai* does their best to learn all they can and gives their *sempai* their attention. The *sempai* does their best to make sure their *kōhai* is learning things quickly so that, in time, they will be able to mentor people themselves.

It is common in Japan for *sempai* to take their juniors out for a meal in the evening. It's not just a way of blowing off steam after a long day; it's a continuation of the lessons of the working day. At this time, *sempai* and *kōhai* have the chance to talk about all sorts of things: love, life, politics, problems at work, as well as their ambitions for the future.

Good managers understand that there is no such thing as "leaving one's problems at home" or indeed "leaving work at work." It is very common for work to start disrupting our family lives, just as it is for family crises or responsibilities to get in the way of our work. By being there for people we work with, especially when they are going through a difficult time, we can practice a central lesson of *chōwa*: making sure we respond as generously as we can in any given situation.

- How could you be a better mentor to people you work with?

- How could you be a better student when you have to learn from other people at work?

*Balancing work and free time* • If you are anything like me, you might find it difficult to give yourself free time. Stepping away from what feels important can be genuinely hard.

What you do with your free time will depend on you and what you like doing. The most important thing to remember when you are managing your free time is to do your best to value both your work time and free time equally.

As I said in Chapter 1, when we come home, we think of relaxation as a form of preparation, part of the stance of mind (*kokoro gamae*) we need to cultivate to face the next day, and the next.

> **Really value your free time.** It may not sound very relaxing, but I have always tried to fill every minute with learning, with doing, with keeping active. My husband, Richard, found this constant need for stimulation and my need to work exhausting. We hit on a compromise. When we do have free time together, we make a plan to do something or see something—for example, to go for a long walk or to visit an interesting museum.
>
> When I thought of free time as "time off," it was a lot harder to give it to myself. For those of you, like me, who find it hard to switch off, you don't have to. Planning what to do with your free time, even if it's reading a book or cooking with your family, will help you value the time you're not working.

## #WeToo—standing up to sexual violence and sex-based discrimination in Japan

#MeToo has been slow to catch on in Japan, a country in which many people have found it too difficult to make a complaint publicly without their words being used against them. Here I'm thinking of young women in the entertainment industry who have been raped and have had to apologize for coming forward to report the rape.[30] Friends of mine tried to take their assailants to court—and ended up being threatened with legal action. Time and time again, women have been taught that, when they speak up about sexual violence, particularly in the workplace, their careers, and even those of their family members, may be threatened.

The #WeToo movement organizers, in an effort to challenge prejudices in Japanese society against victims, set out to reframe the conversation to focus on what each person can do to build workplaces with a zero-tolerance policy on violence and harassment against women. The #WeToo movement is about challenging a culture in which speaking up is difficult. It aims to harness the power of those in the legal profession and the support of industry leaders committed to changing the system. It focuses on transforming the way people talk about sexual violence and harassment in public so that women's stories can be heard.[31]

## Speaking out when it really matters

There's a famous proverb in Japan that relates to making a complaint at work:

臭い物に蓋をする
*kusai mono ni, futa wo suru*
"If it smells bad, put a lid on it."

This is one of the least "wise" sayings Japan has to offer. If people don't speak up, then nothing will ever change. But in Japan, the lesson of this proverb is ingrained, particularly in older people. The pressure not to lose face, to preserve a company's integrity or a superior's reputation, means that people go to great lengths to preserve the status quo.

This fear of speaking up and speaking out is not unique to my country. The fear, and the danger, are very real. If we don't choose our moment carefully, we can end up getting ourselves in trouble, no matter how just our complaint or righteous our cause. At the same time, when it comes to facing up to unfairness, a workplace bully, or a burning injustice—or challenging the way business is done—we don't want to have to stifle feelings of unease. We want our voice to be heard. So here are a few ideas about how, and when, to speak up.

*Inform yourself* • *Chōwa* is about finding out the circumstances of each situation before we act. When we are searching for balance at work, this research will include knowing where our company stands on the issues we care about. If it's a business practice you are challenging, find out why your organization does things in a certain way and whether other ways of doing things have already been considered. Try sounding out a senior member of your team who you trust so you have as much information as possible at your disposal before you act or speak. You may be the only one brave enough to ask certain questions. Many people may feel the same way as you but, for one reason or another, haven't found a way of speaking out or changing things. For many of my friends and the women I work with in Japan, this is the case when it comes to workplace bullying, sexual harassment, and sex-based discrimination. My advice is to meet, talk, and share your experience with others who are also facing the issues you are facing.

For readers looking for a place to read or post stories of everyday sexism in particular, I advise taking a look at the website everydaysexism.com and the associated Twitter account. Some of the stories on this website will be all too familiar, and you may find some stories upsetting. But in a world where many of us feel we cannot share such stories, they can also make us feel a lot less alone.

For readers in Japan, or those who want to find out more about discrimination, sexism, and sexual violence, take a look at the work of journalist Shiori Ito, particularly her documentary *Japan's Secret Shame* (2018).[32]

*Chōwa* teaches us that finding common ground with other people we work with can help us address workplace injustice or poor practice in a constructive way so that workplace harmony starts working for everyone. When proposing change, a new direction, or a new way of doing things—or when voicing a justifiable complaint—the more you've considered others, the more powerful your suggestion will be. A "we" can be a lot more powerful than a "me."

*Ask questions* • A question isn't a complaint. It's an age-old way of expressing dissent and disagreement. Rather than saying "I don't think we should do it that way," try asking "Why do we do it this way?" or "Have we thought about any other ways we could do this?" Of course, some employers will do their best to shrug off such questions. But we usually learn more about our superiors, and teach our colleagues what we may already know, by asking questions first privately, and then, if we aren't satisfied with their answers, a little more publicly.

*Tell the truth* • There are many issues that businesses don't necessarily like talking about, from workplace stress to sex discrimination. This is especially true in Japan. It can be seen as an unwelcome distraction. Business leaders and managers prioritize workplace harmony, a twisted idea of *chōwa* that really means people getting on with their jobs rather than a genuine search for a more balanced workplace.

While similar things happen in workplaces around the world, in Japan certain problems are particularly pronounced. On trains to work in Japan, businessmen will openly read pornography. There have been many cases of men inappropriately touching women, and girls, on the train to work.[33] Until very recently, in one Tokyo medical school, the medical university entrance exam marks were manipulated to ensure that more men than women became doctors.[34]

Businesses may have a culture where sexual assaults go unreported or are hushed up in the interest of workplace harmony: an estimated 95 percent of all sexual assaults in Japan go unreported.[35]

I am telling you this because the preservation of workplace harmony and the status quo allows such abuse to continue. It is a gross misunderstanding of *chōwa*—a harmony that only works for a small minority. The more we tell the truth, the more likely we are to bring real balance to our workplaces.

*Neither the time nor the place* • After my first husband and I separated, I had to spend several difficult months working out exactly what I was going to do. In the end, the answer was right in front of me. I had always loved learning English. I was fascinated by British culture—the etiquette, the class system, the history of British democracy, the suffragettes, and, of course, movies about British culture: my favorite was *My Fair Lady.* I decided to start a language school in Saitama teaching British English (rather than American).

The men I met in my role as the head of the school would openly ask me what I, a young woman, thought I was doing there. Some men would laugh at me. Some would look down uncomfortably. A young woman like me was not expected to be running my own business. I was expected to wear beautiful clothes and serve my husband. I was certainly not supposed to be talking about matters relating to business.

You may have noticed that the popular anime character Hello Kitty, a cute little girl with cat-like features, doesn't have a mouth. This is no coincidence. From my time at school to my time entering the world of work in Japan, it was clear that, like Hello Kitty, I was supposed to be cute and pretty—and silent. This may have improved when I traveled to the UK, but these problems persist in British society too.

When I was running the School for British English in Saitama, I had to attend a monthly meeting for local businesses in the district. I was one of two women in a meeting of around twenty business owners. The other woman in the room ran the local hostess club. After the meeting was over, we were always invited to the hostess club. I always went along, even though it was made clear to me that I wasn't welcome. I would sit among this group of business owners, mostly men aged over sixty, as the young Filipino and Thai women serving them would kneel down before them, pouring their drinks for them, calling them sensei, or "master."

The time and place for this kind of "entertainment" certainly wasn't in a mixed group of business owners. It wasn't the kind of environment that made me feel respected or valued as a fellow business owner. It made me feel humiliated.

I would like to say that my experiences made me stronger; that I learned a lot from running a small business as a woman in Japan. On one level, I did. However, my overwhelming feeling is of being knocked down again and again. Being able to talk about these experiences now feels like a sign that things may be changing, however slowly, for the better.

## *Chōwa* lessons:
## bringing balance to the way we work

**Bringing *chōwa* to your meetings**

- Decide in advance the issues you need to discuss, which issues are worth discussing as a group, and which issues can be resolved more effectively by email or in one-on-one meetings.

- In the meeting, give your attention to the speaker. Respond to direct questions when asked for your opinion.

- When no one has anything further to add, resist the temptation to speak up. Instead, use silence to collect your thoughts and prepare for the next item on the agenda.

**Forging harmonious relationships with clients and colleagues**

- Try not to think of getting to know people as a battle. When we are overeager, especially when we are trying to sell something, we end up forging superficial connections, at best, without actually getting to know the other person. At worst, we can end up really annoying someone if we try to move things forward too early.

- Whether it's a colleague or a client, put in the time to really get to know them. This is the best way to win new business and new friends and form harmonious relationships with others, whether or not you are doing business with people in Japan.

#WeToo

- You only have to type #WeToo into Twitter to see how large the #WeToo conversation is growing. #WeToo is all about improving conditions in the workplace and changing social attitudes toward how sexual harassment, sex-based discrimination, and sexual assault are dealt with, at work and in society.

From Japan to South Korea, Australia to India, as well as here in the UK, #WeToo is about improving the lives of women all over our planet.[36]

8

# Making Bigger Changes

> "Had I not in hours of peace,
> learned to look lightly on life."
> —Ōta Dōkan (1432–1486)[37]

*Chōwa* teaches us to work out what we can do to set people at ease, to go with the flow, to bring a spirit of realism and flexibility to our lives. But harmony isn't something that happens by itself. The search for balance isn't always as simple as accepting things as they are. Some people are happy to accept injustice as simply the way the world works. For them, the state of the world as it is, the prevailing "harmony," works. But when we face discrimination ourselves, or see the suffering of people who are being let down by the way the world is, or the way we are currently doing things, we immediately recognize injustice for what it is: an imbalance that can, and must, be set right.

A big part of making positive changes—at our workplaces, in our families, or in our communities—is listening to what is going on with other people and learning to share their pain as well as their joy. We know what a relief it can be to speak about pain, stress, or discomfort, and to share our feelings about a stressful situation we've been going through. Really listening to others is about giving them this space to unburden. Some of us are driven to do more than this. When it comes to understanding the roots of hatred, or hearing the cries of victims of disasters, we have a responsibility, not only to listen, but to learn. And once we have done our research—the *chō* of *chōwa*—it's up to us to find the strength to act, as individuals and communities. In this chapter, I want to discuss how *chōwa* has inspired my own charity work, first with the Burma Campaign Society and then with the charity I founded, Aid For Japan, which supports orphans of the 2011 Tōhoku earthquake and tsunami. The key lessons in this chapter are:

- **Open yourself up to the pain of others.** Getting involved in helping others and making a difference can start with hearing someone else's story. This can be an act of generosity in itself. *Chōwa* is about sharing the burden of pain with others and, if we can, learning from it.

- **Do your homework and make sure you are prepared.** We've talked about finding our balance with a more active approach to peace—the *wa* of *chōwa*. But before we act, we need to take the time to read up on the issues we plan to get involved in, no matter how much we think we know or how passionate we are about them. *Chōwa* is about using what we have to help, about working together to build better communities. It means making sure we are supported before we help others. It means asking those in need, "How can I help you?" instead of deciding for them.

## "Don't worry about paying me back"

On March 10, 1945, a single bombing raid destroyed over fifteen square miles of the city of Tokyo. Bombs punched through roofs. Some bombs ignited on impact. Others, after a few seconds, threw out napalm, torching Japanese homes, which were made out of the same materials I described when I spoke about my family home—wood, paper, thatch, lightly packed earth. Over 100,000 civilians died. Over 1 million people were left homeless.[38] From outside my grandmother's farm in Musashi, my mother, who was a child at the time, watched Tokyo burn. She remembers the light from the fires, as bright as the midday sun.

As refugees from the bombing raids poured into the countryside, my grandmother said that she wanted to do something to help. Her family didn't have the money to buy new clothes and build new houses for everyone, but she used the resources she had to give them all the relief that she could. Taking regular baths and keeping clean is a luxury that people in Japan rarely take for granted. Particularly after disaster strikes, not being able to have a proper wash can be a source of great distress. Since my mother's family made boxes out of paulownia wood, they cultivated a small forest not far from the house and owned a fairly large outdoor bathtub that could comfortably fit three or four people at a time. My grandmother organized a human chain to fill the bathtub with clean water from the nearby lake, which they heated and poured into the tub. My mother was part of the chain, along with other children from her village. A line of survivors gathered to take a bath, three or four at a time. Sinking into a deep bathtub, up to your shoulders, helps calm the mind, even at the most difficult times. In the warm water, the survivors could take the time to relax, find a moment of calm in the chaos, and talk to one another. They washed themselves, cleaned the soot and chemicals from their skin, and carried on with their journey.

The bombing campaigns, and poor harvests in 1944 and 1945, meant that rationing continued long after the war. It was only people like my grandmother, who grew their own produce, who escaped the worst of it. My grandmother's neighbors, however, didn't own a farm. They had no means of growing or buying their own produce. One day, they came to ask my grandmother for help. They had no money for food. She didn't have money to give them, but she gave them a large bag of rice. "Don't worry about paying me back," she told them. "Please take it as a gift." It was thanks to her that the family survived.

Years later, when my sister started at a new school, she realized that one of her classmates was descended from the same family. I remember her coming home from school and telling us that a girl in her class had thanked her for what our grandmother had done.

My grandmother's generosity was driven by a spirit of *chōwa*, of thinking coolly and calmly about exactly what another person needs to survive, about what would do the most good.

Years later, when I was thinking about starting my own charity, I asked the same question of myself, as well as those I was helping: "What do you need most? What can I do to make sure you have what you most need?"

## Overcoming hatred

Many people get involved with a charity or community action when an issue touches their life. For me, this came when, after I thought I'd found my own personal balance, I had several experiences that left me feeling as vulnerable as I had when I arrived in the UK. They confirmed my worst fears about what people in England really thought about people like me.

Over two decades ago, I was giving a lecture on Japanese culture at a school in Ipswich. After the talk, I was approached by an elderly gentleman who stood up as soon as I had finished speaking. He headed straight to the stage and began to shout at me. He told me that he was a Second World War veteran. He had served in the British army in Myanmar, formerly known as Burma. He had been captured by the Japanese and held in a prisoner-of-war camp. He had been tortured and many of his friends had died in the camp. He told me that he could never, ever forgive my country or my people. "I hate the Japanese," he said.

*Talk about hatred* • The other people at the event came to my defense. They told him I was too young to have been involved. That it wasn't my fault. I told them it was okay, and I was prepared to talk to the man. The more he talked, the more we all started to understand how hurt he was. As he calmed down, he started to grow more emotional. His anger, his frustration at not being heard, began to ebb away. He told us that, after he returned from the war, he had found it impossible to return to civilian life. He had suffered from terrible dreams. At times, he had felt that his own family was against him. He regretted how much of a burden he had been to his wife and children. He no longer saw his family and often felt very lonely. After the trauma of the Japanese prisoner-of-war camp, nothing had ever been the same again for him.

This wasn't my only experience of encountering people who hated who I was—as a Japanese person, or as an immigrant to the UK. I realized that the problem was not going to fix itself. As long as people in my own country didn't understand the reasons for this hatred, and as long as people in Britain weren't given the opportunity to speak to Japanese people, the poison would continue to spread.

*Understand the reasons for hatred* • I wanted to find out more, so I attended a lecture at SOAS University in London. The speaker was a man named Masao Hirakubo. A former army officer who had served in Myanmar during the Second World War, in his retirement, he began to write letters to UK and Japanese army officers who had fought in and around Myanmar. He invited officers to a gathering every year in Coventry Cathedral. The purpose of these meetings was peace, reconciliation, and a chance to understand the reasons for the hatred former soldiers harbored for each other and each other's countries. After hearing him speak, I ended up working for Masao Hirakubo and the Burma Campaign Society for almost ten years.

Mr. Hirakubo joined the Japanese army in 1942 and rose quickly to the rank of lieutenant. He described how he and his comrades had been brainwashed by years of education under the military government and the ideology of the Japanese state. He had found it easy to think of the enemy as less than human. He had never known a single British or American person before meeting them in combat. I only had to think of my own mother back in elementary school—she told me how she and her classmates had sharpened their *naginata* spears to meet American soldiers in a battle to the death—to know how dangerous this ideology had been.

*Forgive your enemies* • Mr. Hirakubo was a very old man by the time I got to know him, so part of my role was to help him travel, carry his bags, organize events, and handle his publicity. There was just me, a British woman named Phillida Purvis, and Mr. Hirakubo himself, so I felt that I was really making a difference. I found the annual events in Coventry Cathedral incredibly moving. The men would meet, shake hands, and say to one another, "Back then, we only thought of doing our duty and fighting for our country. We were good soldiers. Today, we can be friends." The proceedings were overseen by Mr. Hirakubo. He returned every summer to serve a smaller and smaller number of his former comrades and his former enemies.

Today there are very few survivors left. Mr. Hirakubo, at the age of eighty-four, was rewarded an OBE for his reconciliation work. He passed away in his sleep at the age of eighty-eight.[39]

## Helping those who are left alive: Aid For Japan

On March 11, 2011, the Tōhoku region, northeast Japan, was hit by a magnitude 9.0 earthquake. The earthquake and tsunami led to the deaths of around 25,000 people and left over 500,000 people homeless. Over 1,200 children lost at least one parent and over 250 children lost both parents.

On the evening of March 11, I received a call from my daughter. She told me to turn on the television and sent me a link to watch the live newsfeed. We stayed on the phone for some time, watching the footage being repeated over and over. The tide going out. The wave coming in, thick with mud and debris, carrying large boats and storage containers. As the water came in, it dragged down power lines and swept away houses and people: husbands and wives, mothers and fathers, their children.[40]

*Make sure you are ready* • My daughter and I couldn't just drop everything and jump on a plane to Japan. She had a university assignment to finish. I had a translation job I'd just taken on. We resolved to finish our tasks before we did anything. We agreed that we should be as prepared as we could be before we traveled to Tōhoku and got involved.

I strongly suggest, when getting involved in charity work, that you make sure you are in an appropriate place to do so. *Chōwa* is about finding your balance while being mindful of others as well as yourself. Nowhere is this more important than when you are helping other people.

*Know what you want to achieve* • When my daughter and I had watched the news, I thought of the children whose schools had been built on higher ground who had to watch their homes and towns being swept away by the water. My heart went out to these children. I thought of my experience in Japan as a single mother, how terrible it can be in a country where every aspect of society is built around being part of a nuclear family. Being an orphan can be as bad as being a child of a divorced woman (as I know only too well) when it comes to job opportunities or finding a partner later in life.

I resolved to set up a charity to support these children—the orphans of the tsunami. I wanted to do what I could to help educate them, at least until they became adults and could fend for themselves. This was the beginning of my charity, Aid For Japan.

*Do your research* • As well as grappling with the legal and bureaucratic issues involved in setting up a new charity, I was very concerned that we were doing the right thing for these children. I spoke to several charitable and non-profit organizations, as well as university professors both in the UK and in Tōhoku, about my ideas for the charity.

An important part of our research was visiting Tōhoku itself. It wasn't until December 2011 that we made our first visit. We set up visits to three orphanages and visited other children at their homes. On one visit, we sat with the uncle and aunt of a child who had lost her parents, her grandpar-

ents, her sister, and her pet cat in the tsunami. We'll call her
Miki-san.

Miki was playing happily outside in the sun with her
friends. The same sunlight fell on a photo on the mantelpiece.
It was her sister, who had died in the tsunami. She had been
one year younger than Miki. If she had been the same age,
they would have both been safely at school when the wave
came. Instead, Miki was being looked after by her uncle and
aunt, but they had their own children to look after. They were
about to send her to an orphanage. Adoption rates in Japan are
extremely low, so the chances were that Miki would spend at
least the next six years in an orphanage.

> The *chō* character of *chōwa*, as I said, is also present in
> the verb "to research." The first step in bringing any kind
> of meaningful balance to the lives of others is to find out
> as much as you can about their situation, about what they
> need. You also have to work out—like my grandmother did,
> thinking about the resources that were immediately at her
> disposal—what you might be best able to contribute.
>
> Doing your research isn't simply about finding out the
> facts. It's about making sure you understand as much as
> you can about the people you want to help. This might
> involve not just looking at what they need right now, but
> at what they might need a year from now, and ten years or
> more down the line. When asking for advice on what you
> can do, whenever possible, ask the people you are trying

to help. What would make their lives easier? What would reduce their suffering? Put aside any ideas you have about what you think they should be doing.

*Use your community* • I spoke to as many friends and students as I could about my plans for my charity. They had useful questions and speaking to them helped me challenge my ideas and my motives. A student invited me on to a weekend radio program to talk about the tsunami. A few days later, I was contacted by a lawyer who had listened to the show. He and another lawyer offered to give me free legal advice on setting everything up. My students helped me with fundraising activities, and it wasn't long until we had raised enough to begin our work in earnest.

*It's not just about what you've done; it's about what you're going to do next* • Aid For Japan organizes a special summer residential course in Japan. This offers a chance for English volunteers and orphans of the tsunami to interact and have fun together. The courses provide a wide range of activities promoting confidence-building and learning English. Events include team-building exercises, visiting animal shelters, and learning about the cultural differences between the UK and Japan. Many of our international volunteers make lifelong friends. Aid For Japan also runs a home-stay program in which orphans of the tsunami are invited to come and stay in the UK.

But as the children grow up, we don't just want to disappear. We also want to do what we can to help the ongoing recovery process in Tōhoku, a region that has long suffered from discrimination and being ignored by politicians in Tokyo. We want to be part of the changes happening across the region in the wake of the disaster.

Aid For Japan's long-term aims are to help and care for these orphans through a series of initiatives and support programs. This means forgoing the visits and holiday trips in favor of something new. A decade on, many of the children we started working with still have fond memories of their time in the UK. There are few opportunities in Tōhoku for students to travel outside Japan, to gain experience of studying in a foreign country. So we want to start a higher education program that reaches not only the 250 orphans of the disaster, but the Northeast region more widely. We hope to give more and more children the chance to widen their horizons, see the world, and improve their English (one of the greatest drivers of opportunity in Japan). In the spirit of *chōwa*, we have done our best to see the situation for what it is and to adapt our activities to help those we serve as best as we can.[41]

## Being an outsider: the dangers and benefits

There are disadvantages to charity work. When well-meaning but ill-prepared people travel across the world, even with the best intentions, they can end up getting involved in issues they know nothing about. This can be insulting at best, and harmful at worst. We have to keep all of this in mind and, above all, listen to the communities we are helping.

But sometimes being an outsider can have its benefits. I once visited one of the temporary accommodation centers in Tōhoku. It was a sports hall that had been converted into separate sleeping quarters for families. It was very cramped. There was an area where survivors and volunteers could help themselves to tea and coffee. I found myself sitting alone with a woman who, after a few moments, told me, "I lost my three boys in the tsunami." I told her I could not imagine how hard it must be for her. She nodded. Then she started to cry. "Thank you for coming," she said. I said I had done very little, but she shook her head. "It is such a relief to be able to cry in front of you. I don't want to cry in front of the other women. They each lost a child. Even though they know that I lost my boys, I don't want to cry in front of them because I don't want them to think that my pain is greater than theirs. But I can cry with you."

## Helping people with the power of *chōwa*

*Chōwa* was a big part of my attitude to helping people. It gave me a kind of road map for getting involved. I'd like to share these *chōwa* steps with you in the hope that, if you decide to start working to achieve a positive change in your communities, or start working for a charity, you might find them useful.

*Chōwa* lessons:
making bigger changes

**Questions to ask yourself before you start helping others**

• Are you truly ready to do the work you are planning to get involved with? Do you have the time and energy to commit to this work?

• Have you researched the issue, the problem, or the community you want to help as thoroughly as you can? Have you spoken directly to the people you want to help?

• Are you taking full advantage of the network of people you know at work and in your community?

• Have you thought carefully enough about what you want to achieve?

# Part Three

# Balancing What's Most Important

### 第3章

大事な時には調和！

# Food Harmony

> *Itadakimasu.*
> I humbly receive this food.
> —Japanese for "Bon appétit"

What does Japanese food have to do with *chōwa*? With finding your balance? With harmony? The art of traditional Japanese cooking is called *washoku*—using the same *wa* as the *wa* character in *chōwa* which, as well as meaning "peace," can also mean "Japanese" (as in *wafū*, Japanese style, or *wa-fuku*, Japanese clothes). So *washoku* literally means Japanese food. Typical favorites of Japanese cooking include sushi, ramen noodles, Japanese pancakes (*okonomiyaki*), and tempura. But *washoku* refers to so much more than this. It doesn't just mean Japanese food. The other meanings of *wa* are as alive here as they are in the word *chōwa*. Behind the preparation, the presentation, and even the consumption of *washoku* lie skills, knowledge, and tradition that make even a simple meal a deep experience of culture and a lesson in living history—and in balance.

I want to look at the elements of *washoku* that best exemplify *chōwa*. We will focus in particular on the *kaiseki* meal: a multi-course banquet that brings as many as fourteen courses together, where every small ingredient and every detail of decoration have been considered. It's a meditative master class in balance. But it isn't just in haute cuisine, but throughout *washoku* cooking—from cafeteria food to a home-cooked meal for one—that we can see *chōwa* in action. This chapter will discuss these key lessons:

- **Find your balance with *washoku*.** Japanese cooking is a careful balance of the five flavors, five cooking styles, and five colors. In this chapter I'll explain how to incorporate the philosophy of *washoku* into your own cooking. This will prompt you to rethink your relationship with food.

- **Eat in harmony with nature.** Looking especially at *shōjin ryōri*, Buddhist cuisine, we'll look at how *washoku* teaches a deep respect for ingredients, an awareness of the passing seasons, and a commitment to produce as little waste as possible. *Washoku* offers us lessons not only in personal balance, but also in how to find harmony with our communities and the natural world.

## Elements of *washoku*

Food can be a balancing force capable of bringing us back to ourselves, as you'll know if you've ever felt restored after a wholesome home-cooked meal. This is particularly true of *washoku*. One bite of the unique *washoku* blend of textures and flavors is enough to resolve any inner conflict and feel at peace again with the world. *Washoku* food is often rather salty but it's also slightly sweet, perhaps a little bitter, and packed with *umami*. (Umami is originally a Japanese word that literally means "delicious flavor." It is now used widely by food scientists to describe a strong savory flavor, not just of Japanese foods, but a wide range of foods including mushrooms, soy sauce, and fish.) It helps restore our energy levels and it makes us feel, whatever the weather or the time of year, at one with nature.

*Washoku* has an important role to play in many aspects of Japanese culture. Certain meals are served as part of seasonal festivals—such as eating soba noodles on December 31. These are long and thin: when they're broken, we think of "breaking off the year" and starting a new one. *Washoku's* closeness to the rhythms of the natural year is just one reason it has been recognized as an "intangible cultural heritage of humanity" by the United Nations Educational, Scientific, and Cultural Organization (UNESCO). The full set of reasons that *washoku* was recognized by UNESCO are that:

- *washoku* respects the taste of each ingredient

- *washoku* emphasizes the nutritional balance in each meal

- *washoku* uses fresh, seasonal produce

- *washoku* means that chefs prepare meals beautifully, paying careful attention to even small details[42]

As someone who prepares both Japanese and English meals on a regular basis, I can honestly say that the ideas behind *washoku* inform my cooking, whether or not I'm cooking Japanese food. *Chōwa* informs every one of these basic rules for preparing *washoku*. Behind each of these elements of *washoku* is a search for balance: for the right taste, nutritional balance, oneness with the seasons, or the perfect look for each dish. I believe that these elements are universal. Anyone can use them to bring balance to the way they cook.

*Respect the taste of each ingredient* • While the flavors are very simple, Japanese meals respect the taste of each ingredient. Japanese chefs tend to believe that less is more. Nothing is drenched in overpoweringly spicy, garlicky, or sugary sauces. *Washoku* lets the flavors of the fresh ingredients shine. Aiming to draw out the subtle, slightly buttery flavor of a piece of raw salmon, or the earthy taste of a Japanese sweet potato, chefs do their best to go with the natural flavors, not against them. Many *washoku* dishes are based on ordinary vegetables: eggplant, taro root, sweet potato, or *daikon*. Seasonings, toppings, and side dishes play a role in finding the innate balance of a dish—a salty sprinkle of dried bonito flakes playing off the natural sweetness of a Japanese squash, a sour pickle with the saltiness of a fish broth, or the bitter taste of green tea with the deep savory flavor of miso soup—but they are flavors that complement rather than compete.

*Cooking as a search for balance* • Japanese chefs are trained to treat every meal as a balancing act involving five flavors:

1. Bitter—*shibumi*—green tea powder (matcha)

2. Sour—*suppai*—vinegar, pickles

3. Salty—*shoppai*—salt and dry fish flakes

4. Sweet—*amai*—sweet rice wine

5. Savory—*umami*—soy sauce, mushrooms

No recipe can tell you the perfect balance of these flavors. Taste is subjective. But the next time you cook, whether or not you are making Japanese food, try to think a little more consciously about the balance of these flavors. We should think of each meal we prepare as a search for balance of these naturally contradictory flavors; they can be encouraged into a delicate, and not wholly perfect, harmony.[43]

*Bring nutritional balance to every meal* • A basic Japanese meal consists of a soup and three side dishes, plus a bowl of rice. This is known as *ichi-jū-san-sai*, which means "one soup, three dishes."

The main dish will typically be protein (usually fish, rather than meat). The two side dishes may include tofu, carrots, radish, burdock root, or any number of seasonal vegetables or soybean products, typically accompanied by Japanese pickles (*tsukemono*).

You'll notice that there are very few carbohydrates in Japanese food. Carbs are usually in the form of a bowl of white rice with each meal. *Washoku* largely avoids processed ingredients—such as processed meat and cheese—and includes very little sugar. *Washoku* seems, according to some experts, to have something to do with longer life expectancies in Japan. Those who follow a broadly Japanese-inspired diet, high in grains and vegetables with only moderate amounts of meat or fish, have lower rates of obesity and a greater chance of leading a longer, healthier life.

## The *kaiseki* meal: a master class in balance

A few years ago, I organized a tour of Michelin-starred restaurants in Japan for a group of chefs from the UK. I booked the restaurants and acted as an interpreter during the meals. This wasn't merely a case of translating the menu. To truly appreciate a Japanese meal, particularly when you are eating Japanese haute cuisine, *kaiseki*, you definitely need someone who speaks the language. The lessons behind the meal, the origins of the ingredients that make up each dish, the aesthetic choices, like reading a haiku poem or attending a *kabuki* play, require a translator.

*Kaiseki* was developed by tea ceremony practitioners in the sixteenth century. It literally means "bosom stone"—which comes from the fact that Zen monks once placed warm stones in the front of their robes to ward off hunger. *Kaiseki* is a meal of modest simplicity, perhaps unexpectedly simple for Japanese haute cuisine. But for a meal devised by monks, it is unexpectedly lavish. As well as the five flavors, *kaiseki* cooking seeks to balance the five colors of traditional cooking (red, green, yellow, white, and black) and the five senses (smell, taste, touch, sound, and sight). When it comes to appreciating the sense of sight in particular, *kaiseki* is just as much about eating with one's eyes as it is with one's taste buds.

We arrived at the Kikunoi restaurant in Kyoto one April evening, walking from Sanjo station along the bank of the Kamo river. We passed beneath a *shimenawa*—a sacred rope woven from wheat straw—through a simple wooden entrance. After putting our shoes away in the entrance hall, we stepped up onto the wooden floor of the main restaurant. We were led past the kitchen staff, who bowed deeply to us, all wearing pristine white outfits and matching caps, to a large tatami room. The room had a beautiful view out onto a bamboo garden. The only decoration in the room was a print of a powerful waterfall and a sprig of plum blossom in a vase beside the door. Our waitress, dressed in a kimono, calmly opened and closed the sliding *shōji* door. She bowed to our group then introduced the first course, explaining why each element of the dish had been chosen: the seasonal sea bream, the rice, the *nanjo* pickles and the fried *shinko* fish (a delicacy of late spring). She explained the story behind the flowers decorating the long tray, or *hassun*, on which our appetizers were served. Along with the food, she handed out a Zen saying written in beautiful calligraphy in black ink on a piece of traditional Japanese paper.

I did my best to explain everything the waitress said. It was a lot of information. One of the chefs tapped me on the shoulder. "We wouldn't understand this food at all if we didn't have you interpreting," she said.

I think you just have to try this traditional *washoku* banquet for yourself to *see* that *kaiseki* is as much a lesson, a master class in balance, as it is a meal.[44]

*Cook with seasonal produce* • Thinking about what we eat through the lens of *chōwa*, treating each meal as its own search for balance, also helps us tune in more to the cycles of the natural world. Just as we admire the changing flowers in the field as the year grows old, and change what we wear depending on whether it's an autumn day or a summer evening, cooking with seasonal products allows us to think more about what our bodies might need from season to season and from day to day.

In *washoku* cooking, food is prepared to match the changing seasons as closely as possible. Even the way food is cut and presented may have a harmonious connection with the time of year (vegetables cut to resemble fallen cherry blossoms in the spring, or the shape of maple leaves in the autumn, or plum flowers in the winter). Supermarkets will be decorated for the season too. While these are just small nods to nature, gentle reminders of our relationship with the natural world, they are symptoms of a much deeper respect for the changing seasons in *washoku*.

Here are a few inspirations from *washoku* to help you find your balance by cooking with seasonal produce:

- **Seasonal fruits and vegetables.** Following the spirit of *chōwa*, do your research. Which fruits are in season in your country at this time of year? It will help you feel more in tune with the natural world if you eat fruit and vegetables that are in season. It's such a pleasure, for example, to eat wild garlic when I only have to take a walk to find it growing by the roadside. As well as the psychological benefits of tuning in to nature, it is also much more environmentally friendly to eat this way. In Japan, eating imported strawberries in the middle of winter is seen as the peak of wastefulness and overindulgence.

- **Food to keep you cool.** By following the rhythm of the seasons, we can give our bodies exactly what they need all year round. In Japan, we eat salty, protein-rich eel just before the heat of summer. Summer is also the time in Japan for thin *soumen* noodles with ice, dipped in a little soy sauce. Rather than going to an ice-cream van, we visit a street vendor selling slices of watermelon.

- **Food to keep you warm.** In the winter, we eat Japanese pumpkin soup— we would buy one very large pumpkin which would usually make soup for a few days, to have with our evening meal. On the winter solstice, we typically have yuzu fruit with our food. We even fill the bath with yuzu as a special treat, as both a beautiful seasonal decoration and a form of aromatherapy—we find something about the scent of yuzu delightfully warming, and it is good for the skin too.

*Present each meal beautifully* • The moment I landed at Narita Airport with the group of chefs I was escorting around Japan, their education in the aesthetics of Japanese food began. A few hungry members of the group went off to buy a convenience store lunch box, because they were hungry. They were very impressed. The convenience store bento box is beautifully presented, with each item of its balanced offering separated into distinct sections. The food is bright and colorful—the yellow of battered tempura prawns (perfectly crispy and still hot), plump brown mushrooms glazed with a sweet soy and sesame sauce, white sushi rolls with a shock of pink pickled ginger and bright green wasabi and a small Western-style salad of grated carrot, lettuce leaves, and fresh tomato. This minor work of art costs around 450¥ (around $4.20).

> Balance the five colors. White, black, red, green, and yellow—these five colors are present in almost every Japanese meal. But it isn't just about what the meal looks like. Thinking about the five colors helps to improve the nutrition of a meal. Think about a bento box: white rice, a sprinkle of black sesame seeds, a piece of yellow *tamagoyaki* (fried omelette), green edamame, and a bright red pickled plum to finish it off. My partner sometimes jokes about my affection for "beige" English foods, like fish and chips or scrambled egg on toast, but how much are fish and chips improved by mushy peas? And think about how a breakfast is turned into a healthy brunch with a slice of smoked salmon and a mound of spinach. The same goes

for *washoku*. A little dried *nori* seaweed with your rice, or yellow pickles and cherry tomatoes on the side of a plain miso soup, improves the look and the nutritional balance of a *washoku* meal.[45]

## *Chōwa* and eating sustainably

*Washoku* makes me think about continuity and change: the things that have stayed the same, like Japanese culinary tradition, and things that have changed, such as an increase in meat eating during the Meiji period (1868–1912) and the increase of Western-style fast-food outlets in Japan after the Second World War. More than ever, we should all think carefully about how to eat sustainably, ecologically, and in ways that are kinder to both ourselves and to the planet. The history of food in Japan offers several lessons in *chōwa*. It's a history of a country and its people in search of balance with the environment. But it is also a cautionary tale about how balance, once found, may be lost.

Shōjin ryōri—*devote yourself to personal and natural balance* • *Shōjin ryōri* means "devotional cuisine." It was given its name by its inventor, Dōgen, also the founder of Zen Buddhism, who in the thirteenth century was inspired by vegan cuisine in China and introduced this cooking style to Japan. He called it devotional cuisine because he saw it as the best food for preparing one's mind to absorb the teachings of the

Buddha. If we are interested in reducing our impact on the environment, in nonviolence toward living creatures, or simply in eating healthy, balanced meals, then *shōjin ryōri* has a great deal to teach us.

Non-wastefulness. This is an integral principle of *Shōjin ryōri*. Buddhist devotional cuisine will, as far as possible, use every edible part of the ingredient, including, for example, carrot tops and radish peels, which are often used to make the soup that follows the meal. Why not try this yourself the next time you prepare a meal? Rather than throwing away the green ends of spring onions, cut them up and use them for a Japanese miso soup. If you buy Japanese *daikon* to use in a Japanese meal, don't throw away the leaves. You can cut them up to make a Japanese rice seasoning called *furikake*. Simply wash, roughly chop, and sauté the leaves in hot sesame oil and mirin (Japanese rice wine). Add a little sugar and salt to taste. Simmer on a low heat until the sauce is almost gone and you are just left with the leaves, packed with delicious flavor.

Nonviolence. *Shōjin ryōri* is completely vegan, with protein coming from soybean foods like tofu, served with seasonal vegetables and flavored with wild mountain plants. A typical meal might include *abura-age* (fried soybean curd) or, one of my favorites, *natto* (fermented soybeans). Most Japanese people find it very funny to watch visitors to Japan eating *natto* for the first time. It's a bit of an acquired taste, but you should be able to find some at your local Asian supermarket. A Japanese superfood, *natto* has a strong, lip-smacking savory flavor. Each bean you pick up leaves a slightly gooey trail. To avoid making a mess, it is better to mix it into a bowl of sticky white rice.[46]

*Eating animals* • Japan's historical relationship with meat shows *chōwa* in action: a struggle to balance what Japan's rulers wanted, the finite resources at their disposal, and the preferences of ordinary citizens. In the fifth century, people largely existed on a diet of rice, vegetables, and fish. In mountainous Japan, there was very little land for grazing cattle. The arrival of Buddhism, and its principles of non-violence toward living creatures, saw the first nationwide ban on eating meat. Shoguns and local lords seemed to have at least on rare occasions exchanged meat as gifts, however. On these exceptional occasions, the killing and eating of animals was as ceremonial as a martial art.[47]

In the nineteenth century, along with adopting Western clothes and education, Japan's rulers moved toward Western eating styles as part of their drive toward modernization. It took a long time for Japan's people to get over their long-held beliefs about nonviolence to living things, to kill their oxen—who did a splendid job plowing the fields or carrying heavy loads—and to start farming cattle in greater numbers. When the ban on meat was lifted, a protest of Buddhist monks descended on Tokyo. They believed the very soul of Japan was at stake.

Today, it feels as though the monks' suspicions about adopting Western-style eating habits were well founded. Japan is now one of the world's largest importers of meat. Unlike in the Edo era, or indeed the 1960s when Japan was more or less self-sufficient, today Japan is one of the least self-sufficient of all the developed countries when it comes to food. I can't help feeling that, at least when it comes to sustainable food consumption, Japan has lost its balance.[48]

At a time when we all, no matter where we live in the world, need to think more carefully about our balance as a species and as individuals with the natural world, perhaps we should harness the power of *chōwa* to eat more ethically.

Less meat, less impact on the environment. The more meat we demand, the less land we can use for sustainable farming. When it comes to living in harmony with nature, reducing our intake of meat is just as important as saving energy and recycling.

Eating fish more responsibly. *Washoku* favors certain fish at certain times of year. As well as being in tune with tradition, it's important for reducing our impact on the world's oceans. Take a look at the "Good Fish Guide" by the Marine Conservation Society (https://www.mcsuk.org/goodfishguide/search) for more information on more responsible approaches to eating fish.

## *Chōwa* lessons:
## food harmony

**Finding your balance with the power of *washoku***

• To help you on your journey toward balancing the five flavors, five colors, and five styles of cooking, try taking inspiration from these *washoku* combinations:

• Think how much the sweet, slightly bitter taste of broccoli is improved when it's dipped into a dish of salty soy sauce.

• Or think of a charcoal-roasted seabass served with sweet snow peas with the slightly bitter taste of freshly cut, lightly boiled lotus root.

• Or a bowl of white rice, served with a miso soup with Japanese cockles floating in it, and the cheek-smacking sourness of a small *umeboshi* (pickled plum) to finish it off.

**The five flavors of *washoku***

- bitter
- sour
- salty
- sweet
- savory

The five colors of *washoku*

- white
- black
- red
- green
- yellow

The five styles of cooking in *washoku*

- simmered (like a soup or stew)
- fried
- steamed
- roasted
- grilled

*Washoku* also includes many raw foods. While raw is not considered a style of cooking per se, you are likely to be familiar with the Japanese passion for slices of raw fish (sashimi) or raw fish served on top of white rice or in a rice-and-seaweed roll (sushi). Raw fish has many health benefits: it is rich in omega-3 fatty acids and contains high levels of protein.

## 10

# Finding Our Balance with Nature

> "There is evil at work in the land to the west, Prince Ashitaka. It's your fate to go there and see what you can see with eyes unclouded by hate. You may find a way to lift the curse."
>
> —Princess Mononoke (1997)[49]

More and more of our leaders are coming around to the idea that, as a species, finding balance with our natural world requires action. As individuals, we are coming to realize that action, on a personal level, may require more from us than we have so far been told. While many of us have gotten into the habit of reducing our impact on the planet, doing our best to reuse plastic bags, recycle our waste, and reduce our carbon footprint, we are told that our efforts are not enough to reverse the damage that we are doing to the planet. Thinking about how much damage has already been done makes us feel helpless. Thinking about the scale of the challenge that lies ahead makes us feel exhausted.

The power of *chōwa* alone is not enough to save the world. But it might help us enter the right mindset to reconnect with nature. The first step to bringing balance to the natural world is to make sure that we take the time to think about our own deep connection with nature, to realize how fragile its beauty really is. As this chapter will show, thinking about our connection with nature can help change our response to nature, whether it's responding to nature's fleeting beauty or appreciating its immense power and capacity to unleash destruction. *Chōwa* can also help us respond to a crisis with the right level of urgency, without losing sight of our compassion. Our key lessons in this chapter are:

- **Remember that you are nature.** For thousands of years, Japanese traditional culture has been based on the knowledge that we are as much a part of nature as any other animal. I want to use some examples from Edo-era Japan to show how, even in the midst of our busy daily lives, whether we live in a village or a large city, we can be more active in caring for the planet.

- **Commit to bringing *wa* to the natural world.** *Chōwa* allows us to appreciate nature for what it is: both beautiful and powerful, our savior and our destroyer. For better or worse, we are part of its cycles of creation and destruction, its precarious harmony.

## We are nature: lessons in *chōwa* from old Edo

The Edo period (1603–1868) saw the city of Tokyo, then called Edo, grow from a castle town to become the world's largest metropolis.

The Tanaka family has lived in the same area just outside of Tokyo for hundreds of years. My father's samurai ancestors served the man who built old Edo Castle. My mother's family made and restored paulownia wooden furniture, an Edo-era tradition. I've long been fascinated with Edo culture, but the more I hear about our current climate emergency, the more I see in Edo thinking and in the attitudes of my ancestors something I think is worth sharing with others. The Edo mentality can teach us about finding our balance with nature, something we are all starting to worry more about.

*Mono no aware: the fragility of the natural world* • Birdsong in the early morning, the leaves of a tree fluttering outside an office window and the green shadow they cast across a desk, the insects our children proudly come and show us that they have found in the garden. We marvel at our place in the natural world, but we also know that none of these unrepeatable moments will come again. In the Edo era, ordinary people described this feeling as *mono no aware.*

*Mono no aware* (pronounced *a-wa-ray*) can be translated as "an empathy toward all things." *Mono* means "things." *Aware* is a very old expression of surprise, wistfulness, and perhaps even awe. Ordinary citizens in the Edo era received an education in *mono no aware* from artists like Hokusai. His views of Mount Fuji captured the beauty, as well as the sadness, of the natural world, and our place in it. In the background, we can see the great mountain. In the foreground, we see people enjoying themselves, chatting, picnicking, playing music, unaware that time is precious, beneath the fading beauty of the cherry blossoms. *Mono no aware is* a deep sigh, imbued with the sadness of knowing that everything passes. It's a typical *chōwa* balance of the uplifting and the sad, the hopeful and the resigned: nature is beautiful. But everything beautiful will soon be gone.

- Be more than aware of the issues. We are told that we ought to be aware of what's going on when it comes to climate change and threats to biodiversity. But awareness is not enough. I believe we need to know the facts. I also believe that, in the language of *chōwa*, our "research" should be balanced with a more emotional kind of feeling: a sense of *mono no aware*. The sooner we can all start empathizing with the natural world, the sooner we will understand exactly what we stand to lose.

*Mottainai: waste not, want not* • *Mottainai* can be translated literally as "no waste." It is usually used as an exclamation and means "what a waste!"—like leaving shopping you should have refrigerated on the front porch overnight, or when you're letting your partner know that they've thrown away a perfectly good pair of shoes that just needed a repair and a dust down.

*Mottainai* encourages us to make full use of the objects we own. This also includes ensuring they have a long lifespan. It is also a commitment, wherever possible, to repairing rather than replacing things. It's the knowledge, just like with our belongings, that the better we serve them, the better service they will give us.

How would a society in which we always repaired or recycled items, rather than buying new ones, work in practice? After all, many of us live in a consumer society. We like buying new things. Many of our jobs depend on selling them. But Edo-era Japan shows us that modern urban living can be enriched, not impoverished, by reusing and recycling.

## *Mottainai*—lessons in a zero-waste society from old Edo

In the city of Edo, there were countless peddlers, second-hand shops, and small businesses offering to repair your shoes, your paper fan, your old kimono, even your broken bowls and cups. There were mobile libraries stuffed with books to lend or swap with subscribers. An umbrella repairman carried a load of broken umbrellas made of oiled paper and bamboo which he would either repair and return to the owner, or restore and sell again at half price. These people were the oil that made the Edo economy run smoothly. The result was a modern, urban society, closed off from the rest of the world for over 250 years. An urban society that was as close as you could get to zero waste.[50]

*Itadakimasu—expressing gratitude to everyone who put food on the table* • In the Edo era, farmers were seen as the second most important class after the samurai. They produced the most important commodity of all: food. Closely related to the principle of *mottainai* was a desire, both in Edo-era Japan and in modern Japan, to waste as little food as possible. Even leaving a single grain of rice in one's bowl in Japan today is considered rude. *Chōwa* teaches us that a large part of finding our balance is learning how to respond appropriately to the world around us. When it comes to what we eat, it means showing how thankful we are for everyone who played a role in putting food on our table. Today in Japan, when we sit down to eat, we put our hands together and say:

いただきます
*i-ta-da-ki-ma-su*
I humbly receive this food with respect.

A little less formal than a prayer, a little more serious than "bon appétit," saying these words is a way of expressing our gratitude to the farmer who grew the vegetables, the supermarket where we bought the ingredients, and the person who cooked our meal, as well as to the natural world: the sun, the rain, the nutrients in the soil. Wasting food would be a waste of all the effort and resources that went into making our meal. Saying thank you is a way of recognizing our own position in the picture.

- In the spirit of *mottainai*, the next time you are in a restaurant or at a dinner party, practice asking for less, not more, if you don't think you'll be able to eat it all. In Japan, if you don't think you will manage a whole plate of food, or a full-sized portion at a restaurant, or at a school or university cafeteria, it is not uncommon to ask for a smaller portion. At home, if you don't manage to eat everything on your plate, you may return what you can't eat to the pot, rather than simply throw it away, for the family to eat the next day. Out of respect to the farmer, the person who prepared the meal, and the resources themselves, it is important to waste as little as possible.

- Try thinking more actively about *mottainai* in your own home. Try making meals from leftovers in the fridge, buying items that you are going to use soon rather than stockpiling items that will go past their use-by dates before you can use them.

Sho-yoku, chi-soku: *small desire, wise sufficiency* • When it comes to finding our balance with nature, we need to get philosophical to get to the heart of the issue: "don't tackle the things themselves, tackle the desire to buy more things."

小欲知足

*shōyoku, chisoku*

The characters of this saying literally mean "small desire, wise sufficiency." We could translate this as "less desire leads to satisfaction" but it actually works both ways: knowing what it means to have enough can help us fight the powerful force of desire—which on a bad day could be translated as "greed."

The metaphor of a glass that can be seen as half empty or half full is often used to illustrate the difference between pessimists and optimists. But it also serves to show us the difference between satisfaction and greed. Imagine a glass that is half empty. If we crave a full glass, we want twice as much as we already have. Now imagine a glass that is half full. If we're happy with what we already have, we don't crave anything at all.

The more we want, the more dissatisfied we feel. If wanting something leads to dissatisfaction, it's not a huge leap to suggest that, to feel more satisfied with life, we should work on *reducing the things we want to own*. This is different from the idea of minimalism. Tidying up our lives and decluttering may help, but this won't necessarily lead to feeling truly balanced. To do that, we need to think more deeply about our motivation for buying things.

- Tackle the desire itself. Try thinking, "I have exactly what I need." To find our balance in a lasting way, we need to get to the root of our overconsumption, the desire to buy more and more things, to make more and more money. It usually means more and more strain on the environment, and a world more and more out of balance.

Sampōyoshi: *keep the business, the customer, and the environment satisfied* • Like the samurai, who lived by the code of *bushidō* or warrior ethics, the Edo merchant class was also motivated by an ethical code. While merchants may have found themselves at the bottom of the social pecking order, they took their responsibilities to their customers, their businesses, and the urban and natural environment very seriously. This attitude to how they did business can be summarized by the phrase *sampōyoshi*, which means "good in three ways":

- the happiness of the business
- the happiness of its customers
- the happiness of society

I just have to think of the kind of traditional work my mother's family's company did to see how true this was and to see this balanced approach to business in action. They brought the same sort of attitude to their work as their forebears did in old Edo. The wooden chests my mother's family's company made were made from paulownia wood. The wood would darken as time passed, but the color could be recovered by repainting the wood. As the chest wasn't made using metal nails, but wooden bolts, the wood could be shaved down again and again if it got damaged or discolored. Paulownia wood expands when it's humid, so no moisture could get into the chests and damage the clothes or documents inside. Even if a chest were to catch fire—fires were very common in Edo-era Japan, with such dense populations living in wooden and paper structures—while everything else in a house might be lost, the paulownia chest would be spared, a little blackened but intact, the contents safe inside. It would be the first, and the last, chest of its kind you would need to buy.

Today, major companies make similar promises: for example, that this new model is the only phone, tablet, or laptop you will ever need. But companies stopping support for a model or spare parts not being available for older models mean we are encouraged, or forced, to replace our devices. Churning out new model after new model has had a devastating impact on the environment in terms of waste and carbon emissions.[51] But who is benefiting from this? The customer? Society? Or just the company selling the goods?

*Sampōyoshi* may sound idealistic. But many companies founded during the Edo era still thrive today—in fact, over 50,000 companies in Japan are over 150 years old. Compassion for the natural world—and one's customers—is, it seems, genuinely good for business.

*Start thinking long-term* • When the Tōhoku earthquake struck in 2011, few people expected the damage to be as bad, or the wave to be as powerful, as it was. Yet records stored in Taga Castle indicated that there had been a similarly powerful earthquake and tsunami in AD 869. Silt deposited far inland suggested the records were true. This doesn't mean that the power of the Tōhoku earthquake could have been predicted, but what it does show is that we can't simply rely on our eyes and ears, or even on data gathered over the last 100 or 150 years; we have to think about our place in the natural world in the context of the history of our planet. When we rely too much on what has happened in our lifetime, we forget just how powerful nature can be.

Governments can be tempted by short-term solutions to environmental problems. Unfortunately, this has been the case in Japan after the tsunami. Across Tōhoku, local residents have protested against the building of concrete sea walls. They might seem like a good idea to protect villages on the coast. But the people have asked the government to consider the worst-case scenario—a slightly more powerful earthquake or a slightly higher wave would render the walls useless. More radical solutions such as relocating large portions of towns and villages away from the coast may cost more money and require bigger changes, but they may be the best way to save communities in the future. Ironically, a sea wall may, as some communities have argued, prevent residents from seeing a wave as it comes in, so the very thing built to protect them may be responsible for the deaths of their children, or their children's children, who have no idea how terrible it is for a whole community to be swept away and who haven't seen how devastating nature can be.[52]

Short-term solutions can end up blinding us to their long-term consequences. We have no choice but to start thinking long-term.

In fact, the long term may not be quite as long as we think, given what scientists are telling us about how little time we have left to reverse the effects of the current climate crisis. When we think of climate change, even though it has been caused by human action in the relatively recent past, we too often think of something slow, something glacial. But people in Japan are only too aware that the planet can give us sudden, stark reminders of its power. With the increase in extreme weather events worldwide, we may well see human beings having to face up to forces of nature just as powerful, and potentially just as deadly, as an earthquake or a tsunami—flash floods in cities and on the coast, sudden droughts and heat-waves, violent hurricanes. In Japan, we know how powerful nature can be. We need to make sure we respond with the appropriate level of urgency.

*Remember what we stand to lose* • When I was younger, it felt like every day of the year was about finding my balance with nature. Being in tune with nature was simply what it was to be alive.

It's hard to communicate how closely the rhythms of the natural world run alongside the rhythms of everyday life in Japan, and how it feels to live like this.

On March 3 we celebrate Girls' Day—traditionally, Japanese people didn't celebrate individual birthdays but instead we all celebrated together on this special day. We arranged our ceremonial *hina*—intricate dolls of the emperor and empress and their retinue—and ate *sakura mochi* (cherry blossom sweets), in beautiful kimonos. We also made dolls ourselves out of paper and straw, believing that our bad luck would be transferred to the doll. They felt so fragile in our hands but we would place them in little boats and send them sailing down the river, waving our bad luck goodbye.

In April we'd go out walking in the city with my father after he had checked the cherry blossom forecast on the radio to find out the very best time to see them in full bloom.

In May we'd eat *kashiwa mochi*, rice cakes filled with soybean paste and wrapped in an oak leaf (and we learned that oak trees only shed their leaves when new leaves are ready to grow). This was to celebrate Boys' Day. Families who had boys would display *koinobori*—kites shaped like koi carp—in their gardens. They hoped their sons would grow up to be brave and strong, like koi, to swim against the stream.

In June we changed our clothes for the warmer weather, and I helped my mother to air her kimono.

On July 7 we all took part in *Tanabata*, the star festival. We waited anxiously, watching the sky, hoping it wouldn't rain so the star-crossed lovers Orihime and Hikoboshi could be together in the Milky Way on this one day in the year. We decorated bamboo stalks with our wishes or with poetry written on strips of paper in five different colors.

I remember the winter solstice when the color yellow was all around: the last leaves hanging on the trees, decorations in the supermarkets, the yellow squash we ate, baths filled with yuzu.

And I remember the end of the year, when we ate long, thin soba noodles because we wanted our lives to be long like soba.

As the noodles broke, we'd think of breaking off that year and starting the next.

To describe how it felt to be in harmony with nature, I could point to the more musical meaning behind the *chō* character of *chōwa*. I think that doing our best to live in harmony with nature is a little like being a musician and tuning our instrument until, once again, we find a sweet spot and we are in tune with the natural world.

I ask readers to take these lessons from Japan's history very seriously. Japan has spent over a century learning from the West: how to industrialize, how to modernize, how to participate peacefully in a global community. But today, as we look forward, we would also do well to look back: to remember that green cities are not just a dream, but that, 400 years ago, the sustainable city of Edo was once the largest city in the world. To remember that a whole civilization was able to sustain itself by eating almost no meat. To remember that it is possible to live a rich, cultured, sophisticated life that is only enriched further by reminding ourselves, every moment of our life on earth, that we are nature, and nature is us.

## *Chōwa* lessons:
## finding our balance with nature

**Being more than aware of the issues: think *mono no aware***

• You don't have to be a haiku poet to appreciate natural beauty and experience *mono no aware* (sympathy with nature). Composing a simple list is an age-old literary device in Japan. Try it yourself. Try listing things that fill you with joy in nature. Now try listing things that make you feel sad. How about things that make you feel annoyed? Wasps? The irritation of pollen in springtime? That burning sensation when you first come in from the cold on a winter's evening? Making lists and observations is a wonderful, vivid way of finding your balance with the natural world—the good and the bad.[53]

**Doing business in harmony with nature**

• How can the work you do be more *sampōyoshi*? What small changes could you make in your workplace to ensure your product is better for the customer, society, and your business?

- As a consumer, you can play a part in *sampōyoshi*. If fewer of us gave in to the next big marketing campaign run by the world's biggest companies—whether it's for a new piece of technology or a new item of clothing—fewer items would need to be produced (leading to less waste, less exploitation of scarce resources, and a smaller collective impact).[54]

## Tuning in to nature

- When you smell a beautiful flower, hear the wind, or water your garden, do you ever get the sense that the perfume of the flower, the sound of the wind, or the smell of the earth is trying to tell you something?

- When it rains, have you ever thought that the rain was talking to you?

- I think of my students, many of them younger than sixteen, who have been attending strikes and marches to protest against the British government's policy on climate change. To me, it seems like our current government policies are a case of too little, too late. But my students, on the other hand, have started to think in the long term: to imagine not just their future, but their children's futures, when the natural world will likely be in even greater peril. I think it is time we all asked ourselves, "What can I do to support them?"

**11**

# Sharing a Love That Lasts

> "There are hardships, but there are also delights."
> —Japanese proverb

I have been married twice and have shared my life with three long-term partners, and I believe that sharing your life with another person is one of the hardest balances to strike. We have to manage what they expect from us with what we expect from them. We are responsible for their well-being—and expect them to feel the same and to pay us the same attention. But sometimes we wake up and think, "Am I with the right person? Do we understand each other? Is love supposed to feel like this? Is it supposed to be this difficult?"

A romantic relationship is the ultimate act of *chōwa*. In a relationship, two sometimes very different people come together. Two of my partners have been from England, which has led to things being lost in translation. Finding my own balance in a cross-cultural relationship has not always been easy. In my first marriage, my Japanese partner supposedly spoke the same language as me, but sometimes we didn't understand one another at all; we had quite different priorities, values, and ideas about what marital harmony meant. The longer I have lived, the more I've been able to bring something like *chōwa*, an active search for balance, to those who are closest to me. This chapter's key lessons are:

- **Be aware of your differences . . .** We can sometimes be shy about telling another person what we really want, especially our partner. Sometimes, to avoid conflict, we end up staying quiet, keeping to ourselves things that frustrate us about a relationship. But to truly accommodate one another's differences, we must find the courage to share them openly—there's no way to accommodate one another if we aren't prepared to show them who we are. This involves being honest with our partner and revealing things about ourselves that we may find uncomfortable, but also trusting our partner. It is a hard balance to get right.

- **. . . but learn to celebrate them.** Embrace the balancing act that is sharing a loving relationship. The search for balance in a relationship is about creating a harmony of opposites, not a harmony of sameness. *Chōwa* teaches us to accept these differences. When we treat a relationship as its own search for balance, we learn how to better complement each other.

## The best laid plans . . .

From American television, I had some idea of what it was like to go on a date, but I didn't go on a date myself until I was sixteen. We met up outside Shibuya station in Tokyo. After chatting for a few minutes, it began to feel a little awkward. The boy would ask a question. I would do my best to answer. He would nod. Then he would look down at the ground. He would ask another question. Where was the easygoing confidence of the boy who had invited me out three weeks previously? Eventually he looked at his watch. "We should be going," he said. He told me not to worry. He had a plan.

We walked until we arrived at a café, where we had a cup of coffee. Once again he asked me some slightly odd questions, one after another, which I did my best to answer. We had barely been there for fifteen minutes when he checked his watch and asked for the bill. We caught a train to a busy shopping street in Asakusa. I would have been happy to stay there longer, wandering among the stalls, but he checked his watch again and hurried us along. By the time we arrived at a diner for lunch, I was exhausted.

As I sipped on my drink, the boy got up to use the bathroom. He had left his notebook on the table and I couldn't resist taking a look at it. When I flipped through the pages, I saw that he had planned out our schedule for the entire day. He had divided it into five-, ten-, and fifteen-minute intervals. He had also written down ideas for topics of conversation, questions to ask me, and even how he might respond. He only wanted to get it right, I suppose. But this military-style level of planning was not what I had expected.

## The joy of planning ahead for relationship *chōwa*

As I have said more than once in this book, *chōwa* requires us to have an attitude of mindful preparation: to find out all we can about the circumstances before doing what we can to act peacefully, to bring balance to any situation.

The problem, when it comes to relationships, is that the most exciting times when we're falling in love, or enjoying the company of our partner, are when we don't plan everything in minute detail, when we embrace the unpredictable—something my sixteen-year-old boyfriend would have done well to keep in mind—and when we allow ourselves to go with the flow.

When we talk to our friends about harmony in relation to love, we smile. We know that relationships aren't always blissful. We know there's something inherently funny about making sure everything is "just so" on a date. At the same time, I think it's worth thinking consciously about our relationships as something we should spend time mindfully working on—and working at. This is a popular debate on Japanese talk shows, for instance, which cover subjects such as whether or not we should put aside time each week to be intimate with our partner. I also believe that there is something comforting about having a "plan," even if our goal isn't some idealized harmony. We could all learn from this, whether we are meeting someone for the first time or trying to keep the spark alive in a long-term relationship.

- Planning to settle our nerves. Whether it's planning a special anniversary dinner or selecting the perfect place for a first date, making a plan can help to settle our nerves. Relationship *chōwa* means being as thoughtful as we can about the other person, making a mindful effort to put them first, and planning can be a large part of this. We don't need to overdo it, but forward planning can take away our nerves and get us in the mood for romance. What is even better is making plans with your partner. Then you can practice putting each other first while being clear about your own preferences—a tough balance to strike, but one that is crucial in a relationship.

- Planning ahead by tuning in. The best kind of preparation I know, at any stage of a relationship, is always to listen as actively as we can to our partners. It prevents unwelcome surprises if we tune in to how another person is doing. Think of the way I described listening to my daughter coming home, to the differences in the way she might say, "Mum, I'm home." We have to practice doing the same with our partners.

- Planning time to be closer. On the talk shows I mentioned before, younger panelists tend to mock the middle-aged panelists. They advocate setting aside a particular evening each week to spend with their partner. We can fall into routines and rhythms that don't always include making time to be with each other. But planning and spontaneity don't have to be enemies. A little forward planning—deciding together when to have a night in or a weekend away—can help create opportunities for being adventurous and spontaneous, bringing new life to a relationship.

## The origin of love

The concept of love and romance in Japan is very different from the concept of love in the West. Part of this is because Japan closed its borders in the seventeenth century to protect itself from the colonialist expansion of Western powers, including Britain, Spain, and Holland. The closed country policy was in effect for over 200 years (1633–1853). During this time, no Japanese person was allowed to leave the country and no foreigner was allowed to enter (apart from at specially designated trading ports). The Japanese authorities were particularly concerned about the spread of diseases such as smallpox. They were also very concerned about the spread of Christianity. An unintended effect of this enforced closed country policy was that Western concepts of love did not begin to influence the way in which people in Japan thought of romance until after the country reopened its borders in the nineteenth century.

Japan closed its borders not long after the publication of Shakespeare's sonnets and didn't reopen them until after the death of Wordsworth. It was during this period that certain ideas about love took shape, which people in the West now take for granted: love based on personal preference and mutual affection rather than on social expectation; a single partner who is somehow destined for us, who we are "fated" to meet. I have to say that sometimes the Western concept of love strikes me as very idealistic, even unrealiztic. I've always found the Japanese idea of love a little more down to earth.

The love written about in Japanese haikus is a good example. Haikus, while mostly written about nature, are also written on love. Like nature, love changes moment by moment, and when it happens it can feel fleeting, ephemeral. While the characters in haiku poems may seem unfamiliar—wearing *kanzashi* (hairpins) or walking around in a kimono—the way they love seems familiar. A woman stares at her fan, not saying a word. A truce takes place in bed as the couple first touch hands, then feet. A man reflects on the thrill of making love with his wife in broad daylight. These are all timeless topics and could have happened yesterday, not hundreds of years ago. Then there is *shunga*, the popular erotic art form of the Edo era. One picture shows a pair of lovers trying to rip each other's clothes off but being impeded by layers and layers of kimono. We look at the image, thinking maybe they'll no longer be in the mood by the time they have ripped off all those clothes. And we think of our vanity. Underneath the colorful costumes, the two lovers are just people after all.

While Western culture often sees love as a lofty ideal, something sacred, something almost untouchable, Japan has stuck to a rather more practical, grounded impression of love and partnership as something that takes courage to begin, and no small amount of effort to sustain. Love may, at least sometimes, be something that is enjoyed one moment and gone the next. Love, in Japanese culture, can be about taking things one day at a time. So while it might be said that Japan shut itself off from the rich Western tradition of love, the rest of the world also missed out on Japan's unique, unsentimental take on relationships and romance: what it means to desire, to feel jealous, to feel shy, or to lose a love.[55]

## The hardest balance of all

Forming a close relationship with another person is one of the greatest challenges we can take on. In the final section of this chapter, I want to encourage you to think about the foundations of any good relationship as celebrating what makes us different from another person, rather than smoothing over any differences. When you're going through a bad patch in a relationship, you may feel tempted to pretend to yourself and your partner that everything is fine. But it's far better to be honest about your feelings. When we are finding our balance with someone else, our affection for them is hugely important, but so is our ability to communicate honestly with them. We must be able to find out what they need from us, and not forget to ask for what we need from them.

*Understanding differences* • It may be hard to accept but your partner is, at the end of the day, a different person from you.

*Chōwa* teaches us that the foundation of a good relationship, like other aspects of searching for balance, ought to begin with proper research, even if this sounds a little businesslike. In my experience, living in something like balance with someone else starts with someone we can get along with. While there will always be differences between you and your partner, finding someone with whom you have enough in common to build a happy, comfortable life together is very important. I wish someone had told me this earlier in my life. I had to learn it the hard way.

Whether you have been seeing each other for one month or ten years, there will be some differences between you and your partner that will be impossible to correct or change. To some extent, we all have to learn to accept our partners for who they are: how they have been shaped by their upbringing, their friends, their life experiences, including any previous relationships. This is not always easy. We may hear things we didn't at first expect to hear about our partners—at least, not when we met them, when they seemed so transparent, so uncomplicated. But this journey can also be a huge amount of fun. Really trying to tune in to our partners, talking to them about the events that have shaped them, the things they are afraid of, the things they want, the things they are passionate about, can provide an energy that makes the relationship work. When both people are making a conscious effort to understand the differences between them, it helps to knit them closely together.

*Celebrating difference* • Think of the *wa* of *chōwa*, which means active peacemaking. I think this can help us understand what it means to celebrate our differences in relationships—not by compromising (for example, by agreeing to something neither partner really wants to do) but by relishing the tension between two opinions, two strengths, two people.

Celebrating your differences can mean something as small as learning to love the search for balance in each conversation between you, following where little disagreements lead you—or even where bigger arguments can lead—and accepting each other's strongly held views. You don't always have to agree with each other. You can agree to disagree.

> **Put the other person first.** *Chōwa* is an active search for balance—we always have to work at it and remain alert to problems. When we talk about caring for someone, it can feel a little soppy, perhaps even passive. But caring is a verb. We have to do it actively—with caring words, caring attention, caring ways of being at home together and caring ways of keeping in touch when we're apart.

*You don't have to say "I love you"* • We don't really have a way of saying "I love you" in Japanese. There is a verb "to love" (*aishiteiru*) but it sounds a bit unnatural in this context.

愛
*ai*

The character *ai* is high-minded. It's also used to mean love for one's country, *aikoku*. *Ai* feels a bit too serious for many Japanese people. The only time anyone would say *aishiteiru* was if they were proposing marriage or if they were a character in a Japanese melodrama. I think one of the reasons Japanese people find it hard to say "I love you" is that they feel that love should be shown by actions, not by words.

Young people in Japan, like young people in the West, wouldn't talk about whether or not they were "in love" with the handsome boy in class. They would talk about whether or not they "liked" him. Unlike in the West, however, this word *like* (*suki*) covers all bases. It is the kind of like you would use if you fancied a boy in class, but it is also the kind of like you could say, comfortably, after a fantastic second date. It is also the kind of like you could say after you've been living with someone for a decade: "*suki desu*"—"I really like you."

There is something about this straightforward way of expressing how much we like another person that I think we would do well to reintroduce into our adult relationships. If you are looking for any kind of romance or partnership, then, rather than the lofty heights of true love, why not think about whether or not you really like the next person you go on a date with? If you are already in a relationship, allow yourself to think about what you really like about the person you are with. And let them know.

好き
*suki*
As in *anata ga dai suki desu* (I really like you)

Then there's the word *love* in Japan, which is written *ra-bu*. You'll notice the script here is more angular. This is because this is the script reserved for foreign loan words from English. Love or *ra-bu* is what we generally use to talk about the Western concept of love. It is printed on T-shirts, it's discussed in modern novels and newspaper articles, and today it's discussed endlessly by teenagers, who have seen enough Western movies to know what it means (as much as any of us do, anyway).

ラブ
*ra-bu*
Love, as in *ra-bu hoteru* (love hotel)

Love hotels are a popular form of short-stay accommodation in Japan that allow couples a chance to spend a little time exclusively with one another (and not worry about being overheard through the paper-thin walls of a traditional family home). A couple can spend the night there, or just a few hours. Some rooms are simple, but high-end love hotels may boast hot tubs, fantasy scenes, and rooms that cater to any quirk or preference. These are safe spaces for couples to escape their daily routine and treat their relationship a little more like an exciting—even slightly secret—adventure.

*When something isn't right, let your partner know* • One cultural difference between women in Japan and England is the inability of many Japanese women to say what they want in a relationship. In the spirit of *chōwa* in a relationship—doing our homework before doing what we can to act, and responding generously to others—we need to know what our partner is thinking if we are to have any chance of working things out with them. But we also need to take responsibility for saying clearly what we need. *Not saying what we want, or ignoring our needs in a relationship, will not lead to harmony.*

Whether we're in a short-term or a long-term relationship, we can end up doing calculations in our heads, weighing up the balance of the things we are getting and the things we really need. We say that we don't mind *x*, that we can put up with *y*, and that our partner's habit of doing *z* really isn't a problem, because we love them. Take it from me. The little things add up, and I can certainly see them hurting Japanese friends of mine more than my plain-speaking English friends. When we smile and carry on as if everything is fine, we won't magically achieve a state of *chōwa*. That's no way to find balance, with yourself or another person.

> Don't be afraid to ask for what you need . . . When you are in a relationship, the search for balance requires both of you to ask for things that the other person may struggle to give: greater honesty or greater privacy; greater tenderness or a little more space.
>
> . . . but be *realistic*. *Chōwa* requires us to stay in tune with the real world, with people around us. It is possible

that you're asking too much from your relationship. In a world where we are surrounded by images of perfect men and women, it is not just a case of porn giving men unrealistic expectations of their partners and their sex life, but a culture that is built around standards of beauty that are impossible to achieve in everyday life. If you are comparing a partner to a fantasy, the chances are that they will never be good enough and will never match up.

*It's never too late to find the right person* • I have found that living consciously with *chōwa* in mind has meant I take a rather skeptical view of fate and luck. In Japan we sometimes say *ungaii*. *Un* means "fate." *Ungaii* literally means "when fate is good" or "I am lucky." It is true that sometimes things happen in ways we didn't anticipate. But, as I hope I've been encouraging you to think throughout this book, harmony isn't something that just happens to you. You cannot be passive. You must use your senses. Go out and get involved in your own life. It reminds me of an English phrase I'm fond of: "you make your own luck." I think there is something true in this, particularly when it comes to love.

At the same time, good fortune isn't always entirely due to our own efforts; it has a lot to do with others too. I would never have tried online dating if it hadn't been for my daughter's encouragement. She was the one who made my profile and got me set up. When I started talking to the man who would later become my husband, Richard, we both said we hadn't had much luck on these websites. We were both tired of living up to other people's expectations. We arranged to meet.

I arrived dressed in a bright kimono. Even in a city as multicultural as London, walking by the Thames in a kimono still draws attention. It was a good icebreaker. In a way, it was also a good test. I think he was quite pleased to be seen walking around with a Japanese woman wearing a beautiful kimono.

We had agreed to meet by the river and have lunch together, but we ended up nursing our drinks until late in the afternoon. Drinks turned into dinner. It was late when we finally left the pub and went our separate ways. We were both delighted to have spent the day like this. I left our meeting not knowing exactly what lay ahead, but full of hope and optimism for our next meeting.

Today we celebrate our anniversary every year in the same pub. I think about that phrase *ungaii* (it was fate). I think about *chōwa*, and about the universe being arranged in some kind of harmony. Richard and I would never have met without both of us having the experiences that made us who we were. I would never have met Richard if it hadn't been for my daughter, who put together my dating profile.

## *Chōwa* lessons:
### sharing a love that lasts

**If you are looking for someone to love**

• Sharing the search for balance with someone else is one of life's greatest joys, so go out and find your special someone. Whatever is behind you is behind you. Whoever you were in previous relationships is not who you are now. Think of everything you've learned—even things that difficult experiences have taught you. Think of what you might be able to teach someone else, and what they might learn from you. It is never too late to find the right person.[56]

**If you've found them already**

• If you've found them already, tell them how you feel. You don't have to say "I love you"; you can use other words and other ways to describe what they mean to you. Better still, show them! Try making a plan together—to go on holiday, to take up a new hobby together—or share something with them (a secret, a guilty pleasure, a story) that you've always wanted to share.

## 12

## Treasuring Every Meeting

> "Clouds flow by like water."
> —A traditional Japanese Zen saying

I left Japan twenty-five years ago. Whenever I go back, I pay a visit to my tea ceremony teacher, Toshiko-sensei. Whatever it is that has brought me to Japan—a wedding, a holiday, or a funeral—practicing this 400-year-old art gives me a chance to take stock, to find my balance, whatever my state of my mind when I step into the quiet tearoom. The tea ceremony reminds me where I've come from: every small movement in the ceremony, each careful action, is a piece of living history. The tea ceremony reminds us that the present is constantly changing. Yes, some aspects of the tea ceremony remain the same—the cleaning of the utensils, the whisking of the matcha, the sunlight through the windows of the *shōji* screens. But perhaps one of the tines of the whisk is a little bent. Perhaps this tea tastes a little more bitter than the last time. And of course, the sunlight through the paper windows is different from the sunlight the last time we met. What's more, the stillness of mind, the pure quality of attention we try to cultivate in the ceremony, isn't just something we cultivate together in the tearoom. We have to be prepared to bring our practice out into the world; it's as much about lessons in the art of living as in the art of tea. By introducing you to the principles of the tea ceremony, I want to summarize the key lessons in *chōwa* we've learned in this book and share some final thoughts about how you can take *chōwa* with you out into the world.

- **Remember the importance of kindness, balance, and good company.** The tea ceremony teaches us the value of approaching each get-together—of friends, family, or even strangers—with *chōwa* in mind. The principles of the tea ceremony remind us of the lessons of *chōwa*: that thinking about the delicate balance of every meeting, caring for even small items with a spirit of zero waste, and thinking about how we can serve others are not just acts of selflessness, but are intertwined with our personal sense of harmony.

- **One time, one meeting.** Harmony is not a distant ideal. It's the sum of everything that has brought us to this moment, whatever we are doing right now, whoever we are with, whether we are gathered for a celebration or to mourn someone we've lost. The tea ceremony is the refinement of this central teaching of *chōwa*: that we only have now and we only have each other.

## The art of the tea ceremony

The tea ceremony is really very simple. Making the charcoal fire and boiling the water. The gentle, natural cleaning of the items. We listen to the lovely sound of the traditional Japanese kettle over the charcoal fire. We pour the hot water with a bamboo ladle into the cup. We listen as the tea ceremony teacher whisks the matcha with a bamboo whisk.

The longevity of the tea ceremony goes hand in hand with the treatment of the utensils themselves—and the commitment of both students and teachers of the tea ceremony to a few philosophical principles. The principles behind the tea ceremony are what make this ancient art a master class in *chōwa*.

## *Wa kei sei jaku* (harmony, respect, purity, and tranquility)

As I write this, I look up and see, hanging on the wall of my study, a piece of Japanese calligraphy drawn in black ink with a brush. Three of the four characters on this piece of handmade paper were drawn by my friend, a talented practitioner of *shodō*, the art of calligraphy. The first character, the *wa*, the same *wa* as in *chōwa*, was drawn by me. They read:

和　敬　清　寂
*wa　kei　sei　jaku*

*Wa kei sei jaku* are the four principles of tea. Each illustrates a certain aspect of the practice of tea ceremony, as well as the goal of our practice:

> *Wa* (harmony)
> *Kei* (respect)
> *Sei* (purity)
> *Jaku* (tranquility)[57]

In this chapter I ask you to join me on a visit to my tea ceremony teacher's house. In showing you how the ceremony is performed, I hope you'll find it easier to reflect on what the principles of tea can tell us about *chōwa*. Just as students of tea are able to absorb and practice the lessons of the tea ceremony outside the tearoom, we'll consider how to take *chōwa* with us, out of the pages of this book and into the wider world.

## Approaching the teahouse

You and I are walking through the garden of my tea ceremony teacher, Toshiko-sensei. A stream runs through the garden into a small pond. There are one or two piles of leaves where the garden has been cleared. Three leaves are floating on the surface of the pond. We wash our hands in the stream. Using a *hishaku* (wooden dipper), we take a sip of fresh natural water. We clean the dipper for the next guests who will come through the garden, taking a fresh scoop of water and tipping the *hishaku* so the water runs over the handle, back into the stream. Cleaning our hands and rinsing our mouths with water is a symbolic act of purity before we go into the tearoom. It reminds us that we are about to enter a special space.

To enter the main house, we must walk along a winding path of uneven stepping stones. They are far enough apart, and craggy enough, that you worry about losing your footing. You keep your eye on the stones, their rough quality, and the slippery patches of moss, as you step gingerly across, doing your best to keep your balance.

## Wa—harmony between host and guests

When we're talking about the tea ceremony, *wa* refers to the harmony between the host and their guests. *Wa* is about the commitment of the tea ceremony teachers, and their students, to prepare thoroughly for the tea ceremony. As in *chōwa*, preparation and research are the key to a successful, harmonious tea gathering.

For my tea ceremony teacher, preparations begin weeks in advance. Toshiko-sensei sends invitations to her guests, changes the *shōji* paper on the sliding doors, finds out a little about each guest so she can make introductions. She will make sure she clears the garden and, on the morning of the ceremony, together with kitchen staff at the teahouse, she prepares a *kaiseki* meal for us all. She will also make sure she prepares for unforeseen events (she keeps a store of spare accessories for the tea ceremony in case anyone has forgotten theirs).

She never stops smiling. I'm always struck by Toshiko-sensei's kindness. Her reputation in the world of tea is enough to make her intimidating, especially for newcomers. But her smiles help us all relax.

Of course, we, her guests, have made sure that we prepare thoroughly too. We have checked that our kimono is suitable for the occasion, consulted an etiquette book to ensure we have tied the correct knot in our *obi*, and washed our hands and mouths in the garden. This is more a gesture that we are setting aside, if only for a short while, all thoughts of the material world, of the world outside the tearoom.

## *Wa*—harmony in the tearoom

When people ask me if it's stressful to be so focused on getting things exactly right, to be on my best behavior in the tea ceremony, I answer honestly that it's not at all. It is like learning a kind of dance or being on stage. The way we move, the sort of things we might speak about, were all decided over 400 years ago by the tea master Sen no Rikyū. We try to get the gestures right, to the centimeter, as they were performed back then. The tea ceremony allows us to sever our connection to the modern world, to slip back in time to discover another culture's sense of sophistication, education, and conversation. Like performing in a play, we enjoy being an integral part of a group, committing to doing something together and wanting to get things right.

Before the tea-drinking part of the ceremony begins, the tea ceremony teacher presents us with a tray of traditional Japanese sweets. In fact, what first excited me about the tea ceremony was the opportunity to try these lovely sweets—*wagashi*—which are usually made from bean paste. Their sweetness comes from natural fruit, and they're lightly dusted with sugar. The tea ceremony usually takes place after a meal. These sweets are a kind of dessert. After we have eaten the *wagashi*, the ceremony really begins.

*Chōwa* means starting on the right foot by doing our research and being prepared. The tea ceremony requires special equipment, but its lessons about dressing appropriately for the time, place, and occasion, and being as prepared as we can be, even for the worst-case scenario, also apply to our daily lives.

*Chōwa* means cultivating a calm and collected stance of mind. Taking the time to find that place of focus and balance in our mind is the best preparation for the tea ceremony. It is also the best gift we can take with us back to the world outside the tearoom: whether it is being with our families or making sure we treat our colleagues and clients well at work, learning something new or helping other people, practicing *chōwa* stems from, and seeks, this calm stance of mind.

## *Kei*—respect for the utensils

An important part of creating an atmosphere of harmony in the tearoom is the respect and care we show to every item used in the ceremony. No matter how old or how new they are, we treat all items in the tearoom equally. Cleaning each item used in the ceremony is, in a way, just as important as the drinking of tea itself. These are the items we use in the ceremony:

- the container for the tea
- the matcha
- the tea bowl
- the bamboo ladle used to serve the tea
- the bamboo stick used for putting matcha in the cups
- the bamboo whisk for stirring the tea
- a beautiful cloth used to keep these items clean

Once we are all sitting down, Toshiko-sensei bows to us and begins to clean the tea ceremony utensils with the *fukusa* (cloth): first the *natsume* (the container), then the *chawan* (the tea bowl), then the *chasen* (the whisk). When cleaning the whisk, Toshiko-sensei scoops a ladle of hot water into the tea bowl, lifts the whisk with her right hand and stirs the water in the bowl. She brings it up to inspect each tine of the whisk. Warming the whisk first ensures that the tines are soft so they won't break when whisking the matcha later in the ceremony.

*Chōwa* means treating the things we own with a spirit of *mottainai.* Finding our balance is not about buying our way to a harmonious living space or buying the next gadget to shave a few seconds off daily tasks; it's about treating our belongings with the respect they deserve. Our relationship with things is a delicate balance: we must work out how to serve them as best we can so that they in turn can serve us. Commit to a spirit of *mottainai* (non-wastefulness). Think carefully about what you need and what you don't. Use your belongings for as long as possible, repairing and reusing them whenever possible.

## Kei—respect for each other

Imagine that you are sitting cross-legged on the tatami floor of a tearoom along with me and perhaps three other students of tea. We would be sitting in one corner of the room facing my tea ceremony teacher—Toshiko-sensei—who would sit in the other corner of the room, making the tea. Toshiko-sensei would likely introduce you to the other attendees as my student. She would bid you a very warm welcome. You would bow. As you do so, you notice that my fan is on the floor in front of me and my hands are placed just in front of my fan. This use of the fan is the perfect illustration of balance in the tea ceremony. We are respectful of harmony in the group, but also respectful of each other's private, personal spaces.

Everyone has come together for the same reason—to talk about life and art, to show their respect for this ancient ceremony, and to enjoy each other's company. Introductions will be brief but to the point. When she introduces me, Toshiko-sensei may tell the other guests about my charity work. If they want to speak to me afterward about my charity, they can. But there is no pressure, no obligation, for those who don't.

There's no idle chat in the tearoom. It's a place where we admire the art on the walls, appreciate the taste of traditional tea and the pottery out of which we drink it.

The most senior student will receive the tea first, and then pass the *chawan* bowl around the gathering.

*Chōwa* is about the small things we do to create an atmosphere of mutual respect. Take the time to actively listen to other people. Focus on paying attention to what they are saying rather than on your response. Try not to waste too much energy on emotions like anger and frustration, or on feelings of shame and failure. Know that these feelings will come, but know too that, like everything else, they will pass.

## *Sei* (purity)—the appreciation of art and natural beauty

In the tea ceremony, *sei*, or purity, is less about cleanliness than it is about natural beauty, which includes the appreciation of art in the tearoom. The art includes the prints of natural scenes or calligraphy hanging on the wall, the vessels themselves used in the tea ceremony and our own, flowing movements as part of the tea ceremony.

We might appreciate the art—perhaps a print of mountains or a waterfall. We might appreciate the calligraphy, which often reflects a *zengo*, or zen saying. We have already introduced a few throughout the book, such as *shōyoku*, *chi-shoku* (small desire, wise sufficiency), and *kō-un-ryū-sui*—"clouds flow like water" (the *zengo* I used to open this chapter).

Another aspect of appreciating calligraphy is the way it has been drawn. It is said that the way a warrior drew their sword would show you what sort of person they were. It is the same with calligraphy. The way you wield your brush can say a lot about your character. It is very exciting to see the calligraphy of someone important from the past—of samurai, martial artists, actors, or great politicians. Just like when we reread a letter from a childhood friend, we notice that it may have been carefully written—for example, when sharing bad news—or dashed off hastily. Looking at old calligraphy can feel like receiving a personal letter from hundreds of years ago.

When it comes to asking questions about calligraphy, the art on the walls, the flower arrangement in the room, or even the pottery itself—many of the vessels used for tea ceremony are years old—we ask very simple questions: What is the name of the tea? Can you tell us a little about today's flowers? What is the history of the vase?

The important thing about the art in the tearoom, and the tearoom itself, is its quality of *sei*; a purity. There are no electric lights. We can smell the straw tatami. See the floral patterns on our kimonos. The only light in the room comes from sunlight filtering through the *shōji* screens. The only sound is the boiling of the old kettle over the charcoal fire and the sounds of nature—birdsong, or the hum of the cicadas—outside.

*Chōwa* means going with the grain of nature, not against it. Finding our balance in the world has a lot to do with how open we are to appreciating very simple truths: that we are all part of nature. That life involves suffering. That the smallest things are wonderful and have great value.

## Jaku (tranquility)

This word *jaku* means tranquility. It is the same character as *sabi* in *wabi-sabi*. Perhaps the English word *tranquility* hides some of the complexity of this character. It doesn't just mean the feeling you get when looking out at the stillness of Toshiko-sensei's garden in the autumn, but the feeling of loneliness, of melancholy, that comes with it. It's an aesthetic: the kind of feeling you get when you see an old *chawan* tea bowl and know that so many of the people who have drunk from it are no longer with us. It's another of those delicate *chōwa* pairs. It's both beauty and sadness.

The tranquility that comes from the tea ceremony is very similar to the appreciation of the natural world that comes from understanding *mono no aware*—the awareness that everything passes. Nothing continues forever. We must learn to appreciate what we have today, and to value the happiness of others. Like us, they're not here for long. Understanding this truth makes us feel tranquil as we sip our tea quietly, spending time together.

> *Chōwa*, like tranquility, is not a goal in itself. The calligraphy on the wall of my study—*wa kei sei jaku*—is written in a square. This suggests a kind of flow, not a linear journey from A to B. This is because reaching a state of mental stillness—*jaku* or tranquility—is not the end of our practice. It's simply the best frame of mind in which to start implementing the rest of the principles: *wa*, *kei*, and *sei*.

The same goes for *chōwa*. As I hope you've realized, *chōwa* is not an end in itself. While this book has been about finding our balance, that isn't the end of our journey. Our balance is the state of mind from which we can learn to respond more generously to ourselves, keep better company with others, and extend a spirit of active peacemaking to our society.

We never stop practicing *chōwa*—a balance is always a balancing act.

I want to introduce you to one last *zengo*.

---

一期一会
*ichi-go, ichi-e*
*ichi* means "one"
*ichi-go* means "one time"
*ichi-e* means "one meeting"

---

In your life, this moment, this meeting, will only happen once. It will never happen again. This short phrase encourages us to appreciate each moment as it happens.

Where are you reading this book? As you read these words, what other thoughts are going through your head? What does it feel like to listen to my voice in these pages? Think about this moment, wherever you are, whatever else you're doing. Realize that this moment, this instant, of you and I arriving at this point in our conversation, will never come again. We will meet here just once, only to part and continue on our ways.

The tea ceremony is like this. Today we may be sitting with Toshiko-sensei in the tearoom of her house. The utensils we are using may be hundreds of years old and have been used at thousands of similar ceremonies. But this meeting, here and now, has never happened before. Once we leave the tearoom, we know that we may never see them again.

We aren't always thinking about this, but remembering *ichi-go, ichi-e*—one time, one meeting—reminds us why we practice *chōwa*, why harmony with others is so important.

> When you are next at a party, or out with friends, think about your state of mind. If you have been drinking, how does it feel to have had beer or wine? How do you feel after being with certain friends? Or the feeling of heaviness you get when certain friends are not present? Whether you see your friends often or rarely, thinking about each meeting with a spirit of *ichi-go, ichi-e* will allow you to feel the unique balance of each gathering. And to treasure it.[58]

## Life and death

We don't know what tomorrow will bring. In the age of the samurai, the tea ceremony was practiced with the knowledge that anyone in attendance, particularly samurai, could leave the room never to return. A samurai wasn't permitted to take their sword into the tearoom. They had to leave it outside the door in a special place on the wall. After the ceremony, they would take up their sword again. They might head off to do battle in a foreign province where they could die, never again to see the people they shared tea with on that day.

When we look at life through the lens of *chōwa*, we can see that even loss has lessons to teach us about our fragility, as individuals and as societies. Throughout this book, we have talked about how *chōwa* can help us to do the right thing in any given situation. But when it comes to loss, no matter how well prepared we are, no matter how thorough our research, there is no such thing as the most appropriate response, and there is nothing we can do to make up for an absence.

When we lose the people closest to us, it is perfectly natural for us to feel as if we have fallen down, and to feel like there is nothing we can do to get back up.

But *chōwa* reminds us that people come together in times of sadness. It teaches us that it is the people left alive that matter the most, and we must help each other back to our feet.

## The death of Sen no Rikyū

Sen no Rikyū was born in 1522 into an ordinary middle-class Japanese family. Rather than follow his father into business, he pursued a more spiritual life. His study of Zen Buddhism led him to a great interest in tea. In Sen no Rikyū's time, teahouses had become extravagant ways to show off the personal wealth and status of those who commissioned them. Sen no Rikyū's influence changed all this.

Toyotomi Hideyoshi (1537–1598) was the most powerful samurai lord in Japan at the time. He also fancied himself as an aficionado of tea. Hideyoshi was, like many wealthy men, easily swayed by the power of gold, and he commissioned several "golden tearooms." This was quite against the sensibilities of Sen no Rikyū. But Hideyoshi admired the great tea master and asked him to become his tea ceremony teacher. Sen no Rikyū accepted. But as Sen no Rikyū's acclaim grew, Hideyoshi became jealous and even afraid of his tea master. He ended up giving Sen no Rikyū a terrible choice: did he want to be assassinated, or did he want to keep his honor and die by his own sword? Sen no Rikyū chose ritual suicide.

Before his death, he prepared everything, including his own funeral arrangements. He gathered his favorite students together for one final meeting. They ate, read poetry, and took part in the tea ceremony, knowing this would be the last time they enjoyed the company of their master. As he prepared for the end, Sen no Rikyū was able to pass on all he knew and ensure the survival of his art.

When we have a tea ceremony, we still remember with sadness the death of Sen no Rikyū. It helps us understand the foolishness of the powerful, the cruelty of the mighty, and the injustice that this kind and sensitive man suffered. But we also reflect on his honorable death and the thoughtfulness with which he approached the end of his life. It is hard not to admire the strength of mind, the courage, with which this tea master met his end.

Not long ago, I took a pilgrimage to Sen no Rikyū's graveyard. It was very quiet and peaceful, but I was not alone. I was surprised to see a number of people, like me, raking leaves, cleaning his gravestone, taking the time to walk in the graveyard and reflect. I find it wonderful that, over 400 years later, those of us who practice the tea ceremony are still grateful for his teachings.

## My father's funeral

In his final moments, my father thought he heard voices coming from the guest room of his house—the voices of his mother (who died when he was only five years old) and his brother (who had passed away a few years earlier). My father sat down, almost as if to join them, and died.

In a way, Japanese funerals are a little like the tea ceremony. We follow a set of movements decided centuries ago. The atmosphere is tense and solemn as we say goodbye to the person who has died, while keeping company with those who are still alive.

My daughter, my mother, my sister, and I knelt beside the body of my father, who was wrapped in a white cloth, a white veil covering his face.

My mother lit a stick of incense and rang a small bell, which echoed into the silence. After a moment, I did the same.

Sunlight came in through the paper windows. The snow was piled up outside. Gently, my mother told my father that his granddaughter had come home.

My father, the stern man who had passed on to me everything he knew about samurai discipline.

My father, who loved flowers and, like my mother, loved gardening. He had always said, "Like flowers, the best things in life are free." He also said, "A man of flowers can do no wrong." There were a great deal of flowers placed on my father's coffin.

We watched as the undertakers gave my father a bath. My daughter, my mother, my sister, and I gently wiped his face, then stepped back to watch the professionals work.

We dressed him in *tabi* socks and white gloves, tying each item to his ankles and wrists with a small knot. We lifted his body, dressed in a white silk kimono, and placed him in the coffin.

We also placed a pair of sandals, a walking stick, and a hat in the coffin—to keep the snow from his head and the shade from his brow—as he prepared for his final journey.

After the cremation, it fell to us, his family, to place his remains in an urn. My daughter, my mother, my sister, and I picked up each piece of bone with a pair of chopsticks. My daughter, who had never been to a Japanese funeral before, told me afterward that she had felt repulsed, but somehow sacred at the same time.[59]

On the morning after the funeral, my daughter told me she had been woken by a crow landing on the roof of my parents' house. She heard two other crows land on the roof above her, cawing loudly in protest at the unannounced visitor. The crow that had arrived had flown off again. She knew that this was her grandfather telling her to wake up. Her grandmother would say that the spirit of my father may have decided to return to the house to protect the people inside. I'm not sure. But I know that, when we lose someone, we shouldn't be surprised if we find ourselves sensitive to more spiritual things.

## What do the dead eat for breakfast?

When someone dies, when it comes to honoring their memory, doing what they would have wanted, we may find it hard to know what to do. With the living, we can listen, we can look at the expression on their face, we can do what we can to help them feel at ease. We can try to carry the spirit of *chōwa* with us to each encounter. With the dead, we are in the dark.

I'd like to share a short passage my daughter wrote after my father's death. She calls her grandparents *Ojiichan* (grandfather) and *Obaachan* (grandmother), as we do in Japan:

I went into the room where *Ojiichan*'s box of remains were. I opened the shutters. My *Obaachan* lit a candle and a stick of incense. I did the same. I said a prayer. We both looked at the box of remains. We both looked at him. My *Obaachan* said I should give him breakfast.

"What do you give someone who's dead for breakfast?" I asked.

"Toast," she replied, "because that's what he ate when he was alive."

So I went and made some toast and put it on a plate and placed it on the mantel. I looked at it and laughed. It's strange how we have to treat a person who's not there as if they are still there.

When my aunt woke up, she came into the living room. When she saw the toast, she asked me, hesitantly but sharply, "Um . . . why is there toast on the sacred mantel?"

"It's his breakfast," I replied.

"You don't give toast to the dead!" she replied.

"*Obaachan* told me to give him breakfast."

My aunt lowered her voice. "He's the spirit now. You have to give the spirit a bowl of white rice."

I shrugged. "Well, you'll have to take it up with *Obaachan*."

My aunt went to *Obaachan* to explain the ins and outs of what the dead need. I heard my *Obaachan* yell, "He doesn't need fresh white rice!"

My aunt yelled back, "Of course he does, he's the spirit!"[60]

There are no right answers when it comes to grieving. We spend our lives searching for balance, trying to do the most generous thing. But when it comes to loss, we realize there is nothing we can do to ease the pain of losing someone we love. We may all have different ideas of the most fitting thing to do in this situation.

Loss brings us together. When I met the parents of children who died in the 2011 tsunami, people who had lost everything, many of them were filled with a desire to be as helpful as they could to people who were still alive. When I ask some of the young people I work with what they would like to do or be when they are older, many of them say, "I want to find ways to help." Every time I lose someone I love, or hear about the strength others are able to take from loss, it reminds me why I practice *chōwa* and why I do my best to live in harmony with those around me.

**Allow yourself to be comforted.** When we have lost someone, it can be hard to remember what it's like to be with the living. To keep ourselves, and others, from the worst of the pain, we end up switching off the part of ourselves that is usually working hard to live with others. There is no right or wrong way to grieve. But when we are ready, allowing ourselves to receive the kindness of others, to allow them to share even a little of our pain, is an important part of grieving. When we talk about death, we allow ourselves and others to learn from our painful experiences. When we are consoled, we also pass on important lessons. As in the parable of the two pilgrims with which I began this book, the most important part of living in harmony with others is opening ourselves up to their pain as well as their joy.

## *Chōwa* lessons:

## treasure every meeting

Find a quiet place to sit and take a few moments, wherever you are, to contemplate these *zengo*.

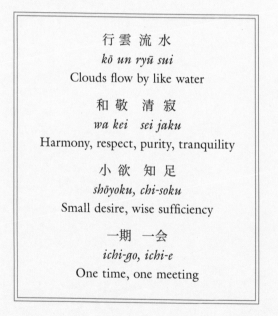

行 雲 流 水

*kō un ryū sui*

Clouds flow by like water

和 敬　清 寂

*wa kei　sei jaku*

Harmony, respect, purity, tranquility

小 欲　知 足

*shōyoku, chi-soku*

Small desire, wise sufficiency

一期　一会

*ichi-go, ichi-e*

One time, one meeting

In the spirit of *chōwa*, why not share some of these *zengo* with others? If thinking about these ideas has helped you find your balance, why not see if you can help others to find theirs?

# Afterword

When I told my friends and students I was turning sixty this year, even though they did their best to be polite—"Akemi-sensei, you don't look sixty"—they still looked at me a little gravely, as if a great tragedy had occurred.

When I told my Japanese friends the same thing, their faces lit up. "Congratulations!" they said. In Japan, turning sixty is a cause for great celebration. In Japan, the calendar year traditionally followed the Chinese astrological system, divided into twelve signs (of the rat, ox, tiger, rabbit, dragon, snake, horse, goat, monkey, rooster, dog, and pig). Many people in

Japan still believe that, when you have been through the twelve calendar years five times—that is, sixty years—you are reborn. It's not uncommon for people to treat turning sixty as a time to start a new profession, go on a pilgrimage, go traveling—to reinvent themselves.

Living our lives mindful of *chōwa* teaches us that the search for balance is an active one, in which we make small changes to bring balance to ourselves and our relationships with others and the natural world.

You may feel like there's nothing you can do about growing older. Wrinkles appear on our faces. We feel aches and pains more deeply. We worry about what we are going to do with the rest of our lives, and about what we will leave behind.

But we need to remember that, as we grow older, we never stop learning. *We grow into acceptance.* This book is about doing what we can to bring balance where we can, but also to accept the natural harmony of the world: the way things are. We have to use our life well, and that means using our energy economically. The more we worry about little things, the angrier we get over trivial matters, the less energy we have to expend when it counts.

There's an expression in Japanese: *shou-ga-nai* or *shikat-ta-ga-nai.* It means "it can't be helped."

We can't change nature. When an earthquake happens and kills hundreds of people, we mourn those we have lost. We also sigh and say *shou-ga-nai.* It literally can't be helped.

It's a hard lesson to learn, but some suffering is part of life. We have no choice but to endure it, to accept it, and learn from it.

**We grow into fearlessness.** When I was a young woman, I would walk into a meeting or a business gathering and I might hear people, especially men, muttering, "What's she doing here?" After my first marriage ended, trying to make my own way in the world, I encountered this a lot. But the more I have experienced this kind of challenge—to my existence, to my own opinions, to my voice—the more hardened I have become in the face of people who would rather I keep my head down, keep out of the way, and stay silent about what matters to me. Now, when I stand in a room in a more sober kimono than I would have chosen in my youth, people do not look down on me anymore. People look into my eyes and see that I've been through a lot. They know I have nothing to prove to anyone. They know I have nothing to fear.

**We grow closer to one another.** *Chōwa* teaches us that bringing balance to our own lives, the lives of our families, our societies, and the natural world requires an active search for peace, a conscious determination to do our research, to find out where we can set things right. We should not treat harmony as something passive, but as something active. Throughout, we have to work with other people.

In Japanese the character for "person" is written like this:

人
*hito*

You may think it looks like a wishbone or the letter n. But this is the character for *person*. It is very simple. Just two lines. Like a little pair of legs. These two simple strokes, unlike the single stroke of the letter I, suggest to me something powerfully *chōwa*.

None of us is alone. We need other people—to help, to find our balance. People depend on one another. Life is about appreciating other people, and finding our own balance is about helping others to find theirs.

I am writing this in my home on a spring day in London. It is the first day of a new era, the era of Reiwa. A new era name is chosen in Japan whenever a new emperor ascends the throne. The name for the era is taken from two characters used in the passage of poetry quoted at the top of this final section ("In a fair month . . ."). Combining two characters from this poem produces the word *Reiwa*. The name of the era offers us a message of hope, referring back to the lovely image of flowers opening after a long winter. It can be translated as "the pursuit of harmony." The name of this new era encourages us—as I hope this book has encouraged you—that now is the time not to expect, maintain, or preserve *chōwa* but to actively chase it: to go out and find *chōwa* for yourself.

It is the first time in over two centuries that a Japanese emperor has abdicated. It feels symbolic to me: an older man, stepping down from the throne and asking his son to take up his mantle. Emperor Naruhito and his wife Empress Masako have spent time studying in England, and their daughter Princess Aiko also studied in England on a short summer program. It is clear they have quite an affection for the country I now call my home. This makes me feel hopeful that a spirit of harmonious partnership will continue between both parts of my life across these two countries, between the nations themselves, as well as between Japan and the wider world.

I am writing this as my charity is about to enter a new phase—helping victims of the tsunami in more everyday ways, doing what we can for the region as a whole, as well as continuing to help the young people we started working with in 2011 to grow and thrive.

I am writing this just months away from marrying my partner, Richard. We are looking forward to our wedding, to our honeymoon in Boston, and to a pilgrimage later this year along the Kumano Kodo trail, deep in the forests of Wakayama.

It is thanks to him that I have written this book. The more I told him about Japanese culture, the more he encouraged me: "You should really write some of this down."

Like luck. Like fate. Like love. We make our own harmony.

# Acknowledgments

I'd like to thank my wonderful agent, Laetitia Rutherford.

I'd also like to thank my editor at Headline Books, Anna Steadman, for all her help and support, as well as the whole team at Headline.

I would also like to thank my husband, Richard Pennington, and my daughter, Rimika Solloway, without whom this book would not have been possible.

# References

Chiba, Fumiko (2017), *Kakeibo: The Japanese Art of Saving Money*. Penguin.

Cliffe, Sheila (2017), *The Social Life of Kimono: Japanese Fashion Past and Present*. Bloomsbury.

Cummings, Alan (2014), *Haiku: Love*. Overlook Press.

Dower, John W. (1986), *War without Mercy: Race and power in the Pacific war*. Pantheon Books.

Dower, John W. (1999), *Embracing Defeat: Japan in the Wake of World War II*. W. W. Norton & Co.

Kempton, Beth (2018), W*abi Sabi: Japanese Wisdom for a Perfectly Imperfect Life*. Piatkus.

Kondo, Marie (2014), *The Life-changing Magic of Tidying Up: The Japanese Art of Decluttering and Organizing*. Penguin Random House.

Lloyd Parry, Richard (2017), *Ghosts of the Tsunami*. Jonathan Cape.

Nitobe, Inazō (1908), *Bushidō, the Soul of Japan*. Kodansha America, Inc.

Rebick, Marcus and Takenaka, Ayumi (2006), *The Changing Japanese Family*. Routledge.

Rosenberger, Nancy R. (ed.) (1992), *Japanese Sense of Self*. Cambridge University Press.

Sasaki, Fumio (2017), *Goodbye, Things: The New Japanese Minimalism*. W. W. Norton & Co.

Shikubu, Murasaki (trans. Royall Tyler) (2003), *The Tale of Genji*. Penguin Classics.

Shōnagon, Sei (trans. Meredith McKinney) (2006), *The Pillow Book*. Penguin.

Stanley-Baker, Joan (2014), *Japanese Art*. Thames & Hudson LTD.

Tanizaki, Jun'ichirō (trans. Thomas Harper and Edward Seidensticker) (2001), *In Praise of Shadows*. Vintage Classics.

Tobin, Joseph (1999), "Japanese pre-schools and the pedagogy of self-hood." In Nancy R. Rosenberger (ed.), *Japanese Sense of Self*. Cambridge University Press.

Tsunoda, Ryūsaku with Goodrich, L. Carrington (1951), *Japan in the Chinese Dynastic Histories: Later Han through Ming Dynasties*. P.D. and I. Perkins.

Zaraska, Marta (2016), *Meathooked: The History and Science of our 2.5-Million-Year Obsession with Meat*. Basic Books.

## Japanese sources

松尾 芭蕉 (1947), 芭蕉俳句全集. 全國書房
　　Bashō, Matsuo (1947), *Bashō haiku zenshū*. Zenkoku Shobō.

佐々木 信綱 (1953),日本古典全書. 朝日新聞社

    Sasaki, Nobutsuna (ed.) (1953), *Nihon koten zensho*. Asahi Shimbunshya.

佐々木 信綱 (1946), 西本願寺本萬葉集. 東京書房古典文庫.

    Sasaki, Nobutsuna (ed.) (1946), *Nishi Honganji-bon Man'yōshū*. Tokyo Shobo Koten Bunko. At: http://jti.lib.virginia.edu/japanese/manyoshu/index.html.

聖徳太子 (604) 十七條憲法

    Shōtoku, Taishi (604), *Jūshichijō kenpō*. At: https://zh.wikisource.org/zh/十七條憲法. English text available at: http://www.duhaime.org.

笹間 良彦 (1995), 復元 江戸生活図鑑. 柏書房

    Sasama, Yoshihiko (1995), *Fukugen edo seikatsu zukan*. Kashiwa Shobō.

石川英輔 (2000), 大江戸えころじー事情. 講談社

    Ishikawa, Eisuke (2000), *O-edo ekoraji jijō*. Kodansha.

## Films

*Akahama Rock'n Roll* [documentary], dir. Haruko Konishi (2015)

*My Fair Lady*, dir. George Cukor (1964)

*Mononoke-hime* (Princess Mononoke), dir. Hayao Miyazaki, Japan (1997)

*Japan's Secret Shame*, dir. Erica Jenkin with Shiori Ito (2018)

*Okuribito* (Departures), dir. Yōjirō Takita (2008)

*Shichinin no samurai* (The Seven Samurai), dir. Akira Kurosawa (1954)

# Notes

All websites accessed July 1, 2019

## Introduction

1 See Nitobe, p. 56, for the passage that inspired my parable.

2 Many of the Japanese to English translations have been made with the help of my trusty electronic dictionary, a Casio Ex-Word Dataplus 8, using the open-source website https://jisho.org (*jisho* means "dictionary' in Japanese) or via the Japanese app for iPhone (version 4.5) by Renzo Inc.

3 A new era name is chosen to mark the ascension of each new emperor to the Chrysanthemum Throne. Japanese era names, like Western calendar years, are used on official documents, calendars, coins, and bank notes. For example, 2019 is also referred to in Japan as Reiwa 1.

4 Source: "New Japan era to be called 'Reiwa,' or pursuing harmony," Mari Yamaguchi for Associated Press (2019). See https://www.apnews.com/bfb2106efca04461a1dd17675a85f18f

5 The English translations of these accounts are from Tsunoda and Goodrich (1951), pp. 8–16.

6 The seventeen-article constitution (*jūshichijō kenpō*) was written in classical Chinese and, according to *The Chronicles of Japan* (*Nihon Shoki*), authored by Prince Shōtoku in 604.

## 1: Opening Doors

7 The Japanese text of this haiku comes from *The Complete Japanese Classics* (1953). This translation is by the author.

8 For more on the history and philosophy of *wabi-sabi*, see Kempton (2018).

9 Tanizaki (2001), p. 4.

10 This meditation is inspired by an online meditation series given by Taigen Shodo Harada Roshi, the abbot of Sogenji monastery in Okayama. A full video of his short introduction to Zen meditation can be found at: https://www.youtube.com /watch?v=LL2XUTeoUsM

11 Strictly speaking, the screens dividing rooms are called *fusuma*. *Shōji*, which have a function in traditional Japanese houses like windows and doors to the outside or to the hallway, are made of thin white rice paper and usually have a grid pattern on them. *Fusuma* are made of thicker, opaque paper. They are used for partitions between rooms and for closet doors.

12 See also Kondo (2014).

13 While serving "the spirit of the toilet" in this way is a popular belief in Japan, it was further popularized by a song by Kana Uemura, "Toilet no Kamisama" (the spirit of the toilet), which was released on July 14, 2010 by King Records and written by Kana Uemura and Hiroshi Yamada.

14 There are several articles about the Shinto roots of Marie Kondo. See e.g. https://www.bustle.com/p/how-shinto-influenced -marie-kondos-konmari-method-of-organizing-15861445

## 2: Playing Our Part

15 For more on *jibun* as "the self-part" and on the Japanese sense of self in general, see Rosenberger (1992).

## 3: Balancing the Books

16 This is the Japanese site for *kakeibo* on the magazine website, Housewife's Friend, which is still going strong: https://www.fujinnotomo.co.jp/other/kakeibo (in Japanese). Books in English about how to keep a *kakeibo* include that by Chiba (2017).

17 See also https://www.bustle.com/p/what-is-kakeibo-i-tried-the -japanese-budgeting-system-to-help-manage-my-finances-heres- what-happened-15909335, https://www.stylist.co.uk/books/ how-to-save-money-kakeibo-japan-career-work-cash/174560 and https://monininja.com/kakeibo-art-saving/

18 See also Sasaki (2017).

## 4: Finding Your Style

19 Japanese text taken from *Bashō* (1947). This translation belongs to the author.

20 For more information, please see "The surprising history of the kimono" at https://daily.jstor.org/the-surprising-history-of-the-kimono/ and Cliffe (2017)

21 See "The Global Impact of Japanese Fashion," with Patricia Mears, Miki Higasa, and Masafumi Monden, moderated by Karin Oen, a lecture given at the Asian Art Museum on 21st March 2019. Available at: https://www.youtube.com/watch?v=kBOeadfaIcw

22 For more in English on dressing according to the season, see http://www.berberoostenbrug.com/kimono-seasons/

23 Source: Stanley-Baker (2014).

24 For more in English on *Tsurotokame* magazine, see Grace Wang (March 2018), "*Tsurutokame* is a fashion magazine for senior citizens in Japan." Available at https://www.stackmagazines.com/photography/tsurutokame-fashion-magazine-senior-citizens-japan/.

## 5: Listening to Others and Knowing Ourselves

25 For more on using mindfulness to respond generously to the world and others, take a look at these talks by Chris Cullen: Compassion (Part 1): https://vimeo.com/25622139 Compassion (Part 2): https://vimeo.com/25642710

## 6: Learning to Learn, Teaching Our Teachers

26 See also Tobin (1999).

27 "The Elderly Education in Japan," The International Longevity

Center, Japan, June 7, 2010. See http://www.ilcjapan.org
/interchangeE/doc/overview_education_1007.pdf

### 7: Bringing Balance to the Way we Work

28 For more information on *chōwa* in the business world, see an
article by Hideki Omiya, Chairman of Mitsubishi Heavy Industries
(2018), "An ancient Japanese idea can teach 21st century
businesses about harmonious partnerships," *Quartz* magazine.
At: https://qz.com/1186023/*chōwa*-an-ancient-japanese
-idea-can-teach-21st-century-businesses-about-harmonious
-partnerships/

29 For more information on NHK's Radio Calisthenics program,
see https://www3.nhk.or.jp/nhkworld/en/tv/japanologyplus
/program-20180904.html

30 Source: Herman, Tamar (10 January 2019), "Member of J-Pop
girl group NGT48 apologizes for discussing assault." At: https://
www.billboard.com/articles/news/international/8518260/day6
-2019-gravity-world-tour-north-american-dates

31 See the #WeToo Japan website for more information (in Japanese
only): https://we-too.jp/

32 There is also a group helping Shiori Ito and those who have faced
similar ordeals in Japan at https://www.opentheblackbox.jp

33 See Brasor, Philip (2018), "Japan struggles to overcome its
groping problem," the *Japan Times*. At: https://www.japantimes
.co.jp/news/2018/03/17/national/media-national/japan
-struggles-overcome-groping-problem/

34 See McCurry, Justin (2018), "Tokyo medical school admits changing results to exclude women." The *Guardian*. At: https://www.theguardian.com/world/2018/aug/08/tokyo-medical-school-admits-changing-results-to-exclude-women

35 Source: https://www.aljazeera.com/indepth/opinion/japan-secret-shame-180726113617684.html

36 New Zealand's Prime Minister Jacinda Ardern voiced her support for #WeToo. See "MeToo must become WeToo," the *Guardian*, 28 November 2018. Available at: https://www.theguardian.com/politics/2018/sep/28/we-are-not-isolated-jacinda-arderns-maiden-speech-to-the-un-rebuts-trump

### 8: Making Bigger Changes

37 The dying words of the warrior poet Ōta Dōkan (taken from Nitobe's *Bushidō* p. 33).

38 See Dower (1986), p. 198.

39 For more, see http://theburmacampaignsociety.org/

40 For more on the tsunami, the earthquake, and the aftermath, see Lloyd Parry (2017).

41 I founded Aid For Japan in 2011 to support the orphans of the tsunami. In the short-term, the charity supports these children and their care givers as they rebuild their lives. Our long-term aim is to care for the orphans through a series of initiatives and support programs. For more information, and to find out how you can get involved, see http://www.aidforjapan.co.uk/

## 9: Food Harmony

42 See here for UNESCO's explanation of why Japanese food or *washoku* has been granted World Heritage status: https://ich .unesco.org/en/RL/washoku-traditional-dietary-cultures-of -the-japanese-notably-for-the-celebration-of-new-year-00869

43 See also https://www.cordonbleu.edu/news/how-to-balance -the-five-flavors/en

44 The restaurant's website is at: http://kikunoi.jp

45 See also Risa Sekiguchi, "The power of five," at: https://www .savoryjapan.com/learn/culture/power.of.five.html

46 See https://savorjapan.com/contents/more-to-savor/shojin -ryori-japans-sophisticated-buddhist-cuisine/

47 See "How Japan went from being an almost entirely vegetarian country to a huge consumer of meat," an excerpt from Zaraska (2016), at https://www.businessinsider.de/how-japan-became -hooked-on-meat-2016-3?r=US&IR=T

48 See Tatiana Gadda and Alexandros Gasparatos, "Tokyo drifts from seafood to meat eating," 9 October 2010, https:// ourworld.unu.edu/en/tokyo-drifts-from-seafood-to-meat-eating. See also Kristi Allen, "Why eating meat was banned in Japan for centuries," 26 April 2019, https://www.atlasobscura.com /articles/japan-meat-ban

## 10: Finding Our Balance with Nature

49 From the Studio Ghibki film *Princess Mononoke* (English version) (2000).

50 The pictures in *Fukugen edo seikatsu zukan* (Kashiwa Shobo, 1995) inspired me to narrate this imagined scene from old Edo.

51 Some estimates suggest that while technology companies were responsible for 1 percent of the global carbon footprint in 2007, this figure is projected to exceed 14 percent by 2040. Source: Lotfi Belkhir and Ahmed Elmeligi (2018), "Assessing ICT global emissions footprint: Trends to 2040 & recommendations," *Journal of Cleaner Production* 177, 448–463.

52 See *Akahama Rock'n Roll*.

53 For inspiration, see *The Pillow Book* by Sei Shonagon, a first-century book of observations by a Japanese lady at court. Her lists include "things of beauty" and "the flowers of trees" as well as "hateful things."

54 For more on *sampōyoshi* and lessons from Edo and modern Japan on living more sustainably, see Junko Edahiro (2017), "Toward a sustainable society—learning from Japan's Edo period and contributing from Asia to the world," at https://www.ishes.org /en/aboutus/biography/writings/2017/writings_id002388.html

## 11: Sharing a Love that Lasts

55 For more haikus about love, I recommend Alan Cummings's book *Haiku Love,* which contains poems from the 1600s up to the present day. It's beautifully illustrated with images from the collection of Japanese paintings and prints in the British Museum.

56 For online dating, I recommend "Guardian Soulmates' (https:// soulmates.theguardian.com/).

## 12: Treasuring Every Meeting

57 For further explanation of everything related to the Japanese tea ceremony, see the Chanoyu website, http://www.chanoyu.com/WaKeiSeiJaku.html

58 For a simple explanation of how to hold a Japanese tea ceremony in your own home, see the Teaologists website, https://teaologists.co.uk/blogs/teaologists-health-habit-blog/how-to-run-a-japanese-tea-ceremony-at-home-the-steps

59 For more on Japanese funeral proceedings, and for a profound but sometimes funny take on the end of life, take a look at the Japanese film *Departures*.

60 This passage, written by my daughter Rimika Solloway, was edited and reproduced with her permission. You can find more of her writing on her blog: http://alackthere.blogspot.com/search

## Afterword

61 The Japanese text is from Nishi Honganji-bon, *Man'yōshū*, Book 5. Japanese text is available at: http://jti.lib.virginia.edu/japanese/manyoshu/index.html. An English translation of the *Man'yōshū* is available at: https://archive.org/details/Manyoshu

# Index

Akemi Tanaka is descended from a family of samurai who fought alongside the fifteenth-century warrior-poet Ōta Dōkan. She grew up in Japan, but now lives in London with her English husband. Akemi is an established cultural communicator on Japan, regularly leading cultural study tours back to her homeland, and giving presentations at schools, universities, and cultural centers. Akemi founded the charity Aid For Japan and was recently given an award by the British government in recognition of her charity work for the orphans of the 2011 tsunami. She is also an expert in tea ceremony, for which she dresses in high traditional costume, and demonstrates this ancient art as a master class in mindfulness and gratitude.

akemitanaka.co.uk